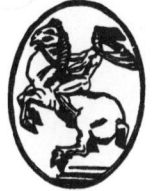

ACTA NEUROCHIRURGICA
SUPPLEMENTUM 22

Alex M. Landolt

Ultrastructure of Human Sella Tumors

Correlations of Clinical Findings and Morphology

SPRINGER-VERLAG

WIEN NEW YORK

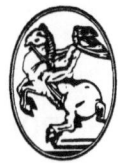

Alex M. Landolt, M.D.

Neurosurgical Clinic, Kantonsspital, University of Zürich
(Head: Prof. Dr. M. G. Yaşargil)

With 94 Figures

Library of Congress Cataloging in Publication Data. Landolt, Alex M 1935 —. Ultrastructure of human sella tumors. (Acta neurochirurgica: Supplementum, 22.) Bibliography: p. 1. Pituitary body-Tumors. I. Title. II. Series. RC280.P5L36. 616.9′92′47. 75–23233.

ISBN-13:978-3-211-81326-3   e-ISBN-13:978-3-7091-8420-2
DOI: 10.1007/978-3-7091-8420-2

Foreword

This monograph on the "Ultrastructure of Human Sella Tumors" is in fact a study of the correlations of clinical findings and morphology. It is a timely and eagerly awaited publication because of the increasing interest of the endocrinologist in pituitary disorders and of the neuro-surgeon in the newest aspects of surgery on pituitary tumors, and also because of the unsatisfactory but still widely accepted classification into eosinophil, basophil and chromophobe pituitary adenomas. This old classification has been mainly based on granule color as seen after hematoxylin-eosin staining, but it does not, after extensive clinical observations, reflect in many instances the type of clinical picture observed.

The author has brilliantly succeeded in demonstrating in a convincing way, by an extensive study of the relevant literature and by his own histological work, that further insight into the biology of the hypophysis and of the pituitary tumor can be obtained only by newer methods of light microscopic staining, immuno-histochemistry and electron microscopy combined with radio-immunological blood hormone determination.

Therefore an earlier diagnosis of primary and recurrent tumors may be obtained which is favoured by the attitude of the electron microscopist who tries to use a functional nomenclature. The basis of the nomenclature is derived mainly from the hormones produced by each cell type. A detailed description of the ultrastructure and reports on special features of the different types of tumors are given, and the correlation between the several histological and ultrastructural features and the secretory activity of the different pituitary adenomas is amply discussed. Under these assumptions, for instance, the old term of chromophobe adenoma as equivalent to "without signs of endocrine activity" is not correct and should be replaced by "endocrine inactive adenoma". In this respect special attention is given to the ultrastructural types of endocrine inactive adenomas such as the onco-cytoma and endocrine inactive adenomas with secretory granules. Also the special features of the cranio-pharyngiomas and of the granular cell tumors of the neurohypophysis are considered in detail.

On the whole, it may be stated that this publication is a landmark in research into correlations of clinical findings and the morphology of the pituitary gland and provides new insights into the biology of the pituitary disorders. Therefore it will be of great benefit to the endocrinologist and neurosurgeon.

HUGO KRAYENBÜHL
Honorary Professor and Former Director
of the Neurosurgical Clinic
of the University of Zürich

Contents

List of Abbreviations Used

ACTH	Adrenocorticotrophic hormone
AMP	Adenosine monophosphate
CRL	Crown rump length
FSH	Follicle stimulating hormone
GH	Growth hormone
HGH	Human growth hormone
LH	Luteinizing hormone
LTH	Luteotrophic hormone, prolactin
RER	Rough surfaced endoplasmic reticulum
-RF	Releasing factor
TSH	Thyroid stimulating hormone

1. Introduction

The tumors of the sella region in man always have been a challenge to pathologists, endocrinologists, and surgeons since the first successful operations for pituitary adenomas performed by Horsley in 1889 (Horsley, 1906), who used the transfrontal and transtemporal approaches and by Schloffer in 1907, who performed the first transnasal intervention. The challenge has been manyfold. For the surgeon it was mainly the formidable localization of the tumors surrounded by a number of important and delicate structures including the cavernous sinus, optic nerves, circle of Willis, and hypothalamus whose damage could mean death or invalidism to the patient. For the clinician it was the bifold symptomatology: 1. neurological signs caused by damage to the cranial nerves located above and lateral to the sella or by compression of the cerebrospinal fluid pathways and 2. signs of increased or decreased endocrinological activity of the adenohypophysis and neurohypophysis. For the pathologist the origin of the neoplasms from all three germinal layers (neuro-ectoderm, entoderm and mesoderm) resulted in a large variety of basically different histological pictures: pituitary adenomas, craniopharyngiomas, meningiomas, and granular cell tumors of the posterior lobe.

Much is known about the biology and classification of the craniopharyngiomas and meningiomas. In spite of an enormous bulk of knowledge concerning the pituitary adenomas, we have to admit that their present classification, which is mainly based on the granule color as seen after hematoxylin-eosin staining, does not reflect the type of clinical picture observed. Acromegaly can be produced by chromophobe as well as by eosinophilic adenomas. The eosinophilic oncocytomas do not show any signs of hormone production.—We will demonstrate in the following chapters that newer methods of light microscopic staining, immunohistochemistry, and electron microscopy present an entirely different picture concerning the relationship of the adenomas with the different endocrinological syndromes observed. These new methods will have to be used in the future to allow further insight into the biology of these tumors. This knowledge, combined with today's methods of radioimmunological blood hormone determination, ultimately will be used for the benefit of the patient by allowing an earlier diagnosis of primary and

recurrent tumors of the adenohypophysis.—The problem of malignant
adenohypophysial tumors is still unsolved since conventional histology
often has failed to demonstrate the characteristics of a pituitary cancer.—
The present knowledge of the granular cell tumors of the neurohypophysis and pituitary stalk is even less advanced. There are still no definite
indications as to whether or not this is a true neoplasm or a thesauris-
mosis.

The following chapters will deal with the results of the ultrastructural
examination of 111 tumors of the sella region. We will try to find rela-
tionships between the morphological findings, the results of the clinical
and endocrinological evaluation and subsequent operative findings. The
literature concerning the ultrastructure of the normal human hypophysis
as well as of the human hypophysial tumors will be reviewed thoroughly.
Reports concerning the light microscopy of human pathological material,
clinical descriptions, and electron microscopy of experimental material
of laboratory animals will be used where necessary. On occasion we will
present the literature concerning light and electron microscopy of the
normal pituitary in mammalians. Material originating from other verte-
brates and invertebrates will not be mentioned.

This monograph could not have been written without the most
generous help of my inspiring teachers and chiefs Prof. Dr. H. Krayenbühl and Prof. Dr. M. G. Yaşargil. They operated on a large number of
the patients presented and focused my interest on the unsolved problems
of pituitary pathology. I thank both for their continuing interest and
support. I also wish to express my gratitude to Prof. Dr. A. Labhart
and Prof. Dr. R. E. Froesch, Department of Internal Medicine, Kantonsspital Zürich, Prof. Dr. A. Prader, Children's Hospital, Zürich, and
numerous internists and ophthalmologists in the vicinity of Zürich for
referring the patients and supplying the clinical data. Prof. Dr. Ch.
Hedinger and Dr. E. Pfenninger, Institute of Pathology, Kantonsspital
Zürich performed the light microscopical examinations and allowed me
to review the slides. Prof. Dr. U. Fisch, Department of Otorhinolaryn-
gology, Kantonsspital Zürich and his collegues participated actively in
the transnasal operations of numerous pituitary tumors. The data of
the radioimmunological hormone determinations were supplied by PD
Dr. R. Illig, Children's Hospital Zürich (HGH), PD Dr. G. Zahnd,
Department of Médicine, Hôpital Cantonal Genève (HGH), Dr. E. del
Pozo, Sandoz AG, Basel (LTH), and PD Dr. J. Girard, Children's Hospital, Basel (ACTH). Dr. O. Friedman and Dr. P. Kelly, Collaborative
Research Inc., Waltham, Mass., USA performed the tissue culture
experiments with some of our pituitary adenomas and supplied the data
concerning the hormone production of these tumors. PD Dr. W. Wegmann, Department of Pathology, Kantonsspital Zürich performed the

electron micrographs of one granular cell tumor. The radiological examinations were done by Prof. Dr. J. Wellauer, Department of Diagnostic Radiology, Kantonsspital Zürich and Dr. H. Etter, Department of Radiology, Kantonsspital Luzern (Fig. 92). Prof. Dr. K. Bauknecht and Dipl. math. A. Leuzinger, Institute for Informatics, University of Zürich performed the mathematical evaluation of the granule size distribution curves.

The book could not have been written without the continuous help of Dr. B. Zumstein, Mrs. H. U. Hosbach-Züst Dipl. zool., and Mrs. U. Ryffel-Gysin Dipl. zool. who did the largest part of the technical work presented. I thank them for their cooperation as well as Dr. J. L. Fox, Washington D.C., USA, Dr. Sidney S. Schochet, Galveston, Texas, USA, Mrs. M. Steiner, and Miss A. Stutz, for their inestimable help in translating and editing the manuscript.

2. Material and Methods

This report is based on the results of the ultrastructural examination of 114 biopsies of various tumors of the sella region of 111 patients. All tumors have been operated on in the Department of Neurological Surgery of the Kantonsspital Zürich in almost equal numbers by Prof. H. Krayenbühl, Prof. M. G. Yaşargil, and the author in the years 1971 through 1973; a few also were operated on in the years 1969, 1970 and 1974. The

Table 1. *Histological and Clinical Diagnosis of the Cases Presented*

Pituitary adenomas	
Endocrine inactive adenomas	49
Acromegaly	29
Forbes-Albright syndrome	4
Oncocytoma	4
Cysts	2
Nelson's syndrome	2
Cushing's syndrome	1
Addison's disease	1
Craniopharyngiomas	16
Granular cell myoblastomas	2
Intrasellar meningioma	1
Total	111 patients

exact type of the specimens examined is indicated in Table 1.—About two thirds of the pituitary adenomas were operated on by the transsphenoidal approach and the remaining third by the transfrontal or transfronto-temporal approach. The transcranial route was used in all but one craniopharyngioma which was almost entirely situated within the sella and therefore was removed from below. One granular cell tumor and the intrasellar meningioma were operated on from above. The tissue of the second granular cell tumor was obtained from autopsy.

The tumor biopsies always were removed shortly after the first contact with the tumor and after coagulation and incision of the overlying dura or capsule. Tumor particles with a diameter of 5 mm were immersed within less than 30 seconds into the fixation fluid. A further dissection into pieces of 1 mm³ was performed within the fixation fluid. The whole procedure was done in the operating theater in order to secure an optimum fixation quality.—The following procedures of fixation, embedding, and staining were used:

1. Fixation in ice cold 2% osmium tetroxide in S-collidine buffer (pH 7.4), dehydration in acetone, embedding in Durcupan® (Fluka AG,

Buchs, Switzerland) (similar to araldite), staining of ultrathin sections with uranyl acetate (Watson, 1958) and lead citrate (Reynolds, 1963).

2. Fixation in ice cold 3% glutaraldehyde in 0.1 M phosphate buffer (pH 7.3), rinsing over night in equal mixture of 0.2 M phosphate buffer and 0.4 M sucrose, second fixation in 2% osmium tetroxide and following procedures as above.

3. Fixation in ice cold 3% glutaraldehyde in 0.1 M phosphate buffer (pH 7.3), dehydration in acetone and direct embedding as above.

4. Fixation in ice cold 3% glutaraldehyde, rinsing in 0.1 M phosphate buffer (pH 7.3), block staining with 0.1% ethidium bromide (2,7-diamino-10-ethyl-9-phenyl-phenantridium bromide "Sigma") for 12 hours at temperature 4 °C, washing with multiple changes of distilled water for 12–24 hours, dehydration in acetone, embedding in Durcupan and staining of ultrathin sections with uranyl acetate and lead citrate.

5. Block staining of osmium fixed material with 1% phosphotungstic acid (PTA) (Gray, 1964) in absolute acetone prior to embedding in Durcupan®. No staining of ultrathin sections.

6. Fixation in 5% potassium permanganate (Luft, 1956), embedding in Epon, incubation of ultrathin sections in 2% RNAse (Fluka) in veronal acetate buffer (pH 7.3, temperature 37 °C), staining in 5% uranyl acetate in distilled water (Yosuyanagi, 1960; Yosuyanagi and Guerrier, 1965).

7. Fixation in 4% p-formaldehyde in 0.1 M phosphate buffer (pH 7.3) for 1 hour, washing over night in phosphate buffer, impregnation for 1 hour, with 10% dimethyl sulfoxide (Nakane, 1970), freeze-sectioning at 20–30 μ thickness, washing in phosphate buffer, incubation for 5 minutes in 0.1% trypsin, and 1% RNAse or 1% DNAse for 2 hours, fixation in osmium tetroxide, and embedding as above.

8. Subsequent single ultrathin sections of osmium fixed material were placed on one hole copper grids covered with a carbon coated Parlodion film. Incubation in 20% perchloric acid at temperature 60 °C (Douglas, 1970) for 8 hours, staining in uranyl acetate and lead citrate.

9. Ultrathin sections of glutaraldehyde fixed and Durcupan embedded tissue were placed on gold grids. Rinsing in twice quartz-distilled water for 3–5 hours, hydrolysis in 5 N HCl, washing in twice quartz-distilled water, incubation in 0.5 ml 5% silver nitrate, 9.5 ml 3% methenamine, 2 ml 3% sodium borate (pH adjusted with 1 N NaOH to 8.1), and 8 ml twice quartz-distilled water freshly mixed for each experiment, rinsing in incubation medium without silver nitrate and four times in distilled water, light counterstaining with uranyl acetate (Peters and Giese, 1970, 1971).

10. Fixation in formalin-picric acid (Nakane, 1971), dehydration in alcohol, embedding in a mixture of 5 ml hydroxiethylmethacrylate (GMA)

(Fluka), 5 ml butylmethacrylate (BMA) (Fluka) using 90 mg α,α'-azo-
diisobutyronitrile as a catalyst and prepolymerization in order to decrease
erratic polymerization (Luft, 1973), final polymerization at temperature
4 °C under ultraviolet light (366 nm). Staining of ultrathin sections with
osmium tetroxide and uranyl acetate.

The ultrathin sections were obtained with a LKB-Ultrotome II
equipped with glass or diamond knives. The preparations were examined

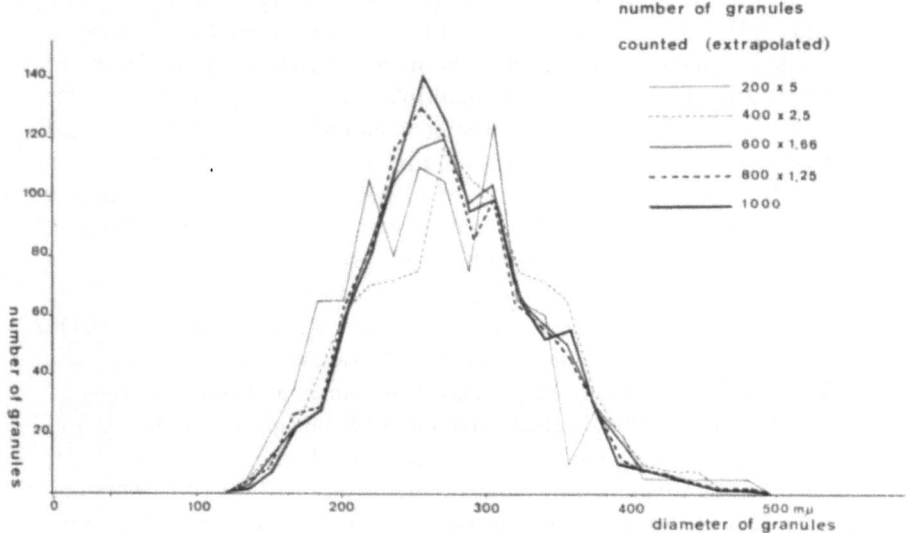

Fig. 1. Granule size distribution curves resulting from measuring and
extrapolating 200, 400, 600, 800, and 1000 secretory granules in a case of
acromegaly

with a Philips electron microscope EM 300 using an acceleration voltage
of 60 kV and 50 μ objective apertures.

A number of forty to 120 micrographs from individual cases obtained
at the same magnification were used for the determination of the granule
size distribution curves. A grating replica was photographed at the
beginning and end of each film. The magnification of the electron
microscope was not changed during the whole procedure. The negatives
were enlarged six times to a final magnification of × 35,600 which was
calibrated with the grating replica. The granules were measured and
counted with the semiautomatic particle size analyzer (TGZ 3, Zeiss)
described by Endter and Gebauer (1956). Fig. 1 shows the comparison
of the size distribution curves resulting from measurements of 200, 400,
600, 800, and 1,000 granules of the same case. It can be seen that the

curves resulting from the evaluation of 600, 800, and 1,000 granules are almost identical. Therefore we have tried to obtain measurements of at least 500 granules in each case. One thousand were counted in the large majority of the examples presented. Histograms were drawn from the data obtained. The average particle size and the standard deviation of the curves were calculated with a programmable desk calculator (Hewlett-Packard A 98 20) at the same time.

3. Ultrastructure of the Normal Pituitary

The first important step in differentiation of the adenohypophysial cell types was made by Schönemann (1892). He described eosinophilic, cyanophilic (basophilic), and chromophobe elements. The system of three cell types was used with minor modifications until Romeis (1940) published his fundamental study concerning the histology of the pituitary gland. He counted five different granulated, one undifferentiated, and one vacuolated, exhausted cell types. Pathologists and clinicans have continued to use the old, three cell type system in spite of these new histological results. This mainly was due to the fact that the "kresazan-method" of Romeis was quite capricious and produced unreliable results in unskilled hands. A large variety of fixation and staining methods was developed because of these difficulties (for review see Herlant, 1964; Purves, 1966). Most of these methods were used in different laboratory animals. The use of an almost endless variety of such techniques made the comparison of the results of different authors extremely difficult. Moreover, in some species a certain fixation and staining method may make it possible to distinguish between certain cell types, whereas the same technique may fail to show these cell types in other species.

Many authors have tried to overcome such difficulties by using a functional nomenclature in which the staining reaction was of minor importance. This nomenclature, however, is based, if properly applied, on much experimental work and therefore has less practical meaning for those who use cytology as an auxiliary method in other examinations. Some authors have tried to avoid the laborious experimental work by assuming that if a cell type showing a certain staining reaction produces a certain hormone in one species, it will have the same function in another species if the staining reactions are the same. Many authors have used the Greek letter nomenclature of Romeis (1940) for a number of different species not realizing that Romeis based his terminology on the results obtained only from human material. A great deal of confusion concerning the functional properties, staining reactions, and different nomenclatures arose from this. A number of internationally known cytologists then attempted to eliminate these differences at a conference held in Paris in 1963 (Benoit and Da Lage, 1963). No unanimous solution was found.

Taking advantage of the experiences of light microscopy the electron microscopists from the beginning tried to use a functional nomenclature. This nomenclature was derived mainly from the hormones produced by each cell type. Only one or two cell types could not be related to certain hormones. The electron microscopists took advantage of the fact that all pituitary hormones were identified at this time. In addition to that the ultrastructure of the hormone granules themselves and not an indirect staining reaction, can be visualized with the electron microscope. Variations of fixation, embedding, and staining techniques seem to cause much less variation than different techniques in light microscopy.

Fernandez-Moràn and Luft (1949) were the first to study the ultrastructure of the anterior pituitary. They used the replica-adhesion technique on cell smears of the rat adenohypophysis and found that the cytoplasm of the cells consisted predominantly of distinctly outlined spherical bodies of 30–300 mμ in diameter. They seemed to contain even smaller spherical granules that were embedded in a particulate, submicroscopic ground substance. The differences among the three cell types (basophilic, eosinophilic, and chromophobe) seemed to be of a quantitative nature involving the size and distribution of the granular bodies. No basic differences were found. When sectioning methods became practical, Rinehart and Farquhar (1953) identified the two chromophilic cell classes more clearly. The eosinophilic cells demonstrated phases of hormone synthesis, hormone accumulation, and hormone secretion. The granules showed a diameter of about 350 mμ. The basophilic cells had an analogous cell cycle and smaller granules with a diameter of about 140–200 mμ. A third, small cell type had stellate outlines and did not contain any granules. Most of the following studies elucidating the nature of the individual pituitary cell types were performed on rat material as cited in the two papers above.

Further studies by the same authors provided a better insight into the characteristics of the cells producing the individual hormones. The examination of castrated rat pituitaries showed cytological changes in two basophilic cell forms consisting of formation of empty vacuoles, decreased number of granules, enlargement of the Golgi structures, and increased number of mitochondria. The cells were supposed to represent FSH and LH producing elements (Farquhar and Rinehart 1954a, 1955). A further study showed similar changes after thyroidectomy in small polygonal cells containing tiny granules (diameter 140 mμ). The cells were identified as TSH producing elements (Farquhar and Rinehart, 1954b). The ultrastructural differences between prolactin (LTH) and growth hormone (GH or STH) producing cells in the rat were described in a further paper (Hedinger and Farquhar, 1957). The LTH cells contained the largest granules of all pituitary cells reaching a diameter of 700 mμ whereas the GH cell granules measured only up to 350 mμ in diameter. Farquhar and collaborators therefore have presented the ultrastructural basis of the one cell—one hormone theory which indicates that each hormone is produced by one specialized cell type that can be identified with appropriate histological techniques. This theory fitted perfectly to the cell classification of Romeis (1940) who had tried to

establish certain functional correlations. He had to use the old eosino-
philic-basophilic-chromophobe nomenclature since all deductions were
made from pathological material of other authors. Green and van Breemen
(1955) were able to differentiate only eosinophilic and basophilic cells in
their electron micrographs. They concluded that the five cell types of
Romeis (1940) were artificial. The identification of corticotrophs was
achieved by Herlant (Herlant, 1963; Herlant and Klasterky, 1963). He
described cells with erythrosine positive granules that had a diameter of
150 mμ in his electron micrographs. Farquhar had attributed the ACTH
production to non-granulated cells with stellate outlines.

The first investigations dealing with cell type identification were
based on physiological studies and subsequent examination with light
microscopy since no specific stains for the different hormones were
known. The cytological changes were examined after extirpation of the
end organs (e.g. thyroid, gonads, adrenals) or after treatment with the
hormones of the glands mentioned. Other papers were based on the
examination of the physiological changes occurring during the menstrual
cycle, pregnancy, or lactation. The results of these types of localization
studies have been published in a number of review papers dealing with
light and electron microscopy of the pituitary cytology in various animals (Barnes, 1962, 1963; Cardell, 1963; Costoff, 1973; Farquhar, 1971;
Fawcett et. al., 1969; Foster, 1971; Green, 1966a; Heath, 1970; Herlant,
1963, 1964, 1965; Kracht, 1957; Purves, 1966; Salazar, 1963; Wittkowski,
1971). A specific demonstration of the different hormones can be achieved
with immunohistological methods. Immunofluorescent methods (Lenz-
noff, 1960; Marshall, 1951; Nayak et al., 1968; Rennels, 1963; Pearse
and van Noorden, 1963; Stokes and Boda, 1968) as well as peroxidase
labelled antibodies (Baker and Yu, 1971; Nakane, 1968; Nakane and
Pierce, 1966; Phifer et al., 1973) have been used in light microscopy.
Different immunological methods have been adapted successfully to
electron microscopy (for review see Sternberger, 1967). Peroxidase
(Kawarai and Nakane, 1968; Moriarty and Halmi, 1972; Moriarty et al.,
1973; Nakane, 1968, 1971; Nakane and Pierce, 1967) or ferritin (Tani
et al., 1969) can be used as markers for the reactive immunoglobulins.
The immunohistological methods share the disadvantage that they cannot be used in routine work since the antibodies used are only available
in some highly specialized laboratories. Further identification of cells
and their secretory granules was achieved by various separation methods.
A two-to-three fold enrichment of different cell types could be obtained
by sedimentation at unit gravity (Hymer et al., 1972, 1973; Llyoyd and
McShan, 1973). The secretory granules of some cell types could be
separated after homogenization of the tissue by filtration through milli-
pore filters with various pore diameters (McShan, 1965).

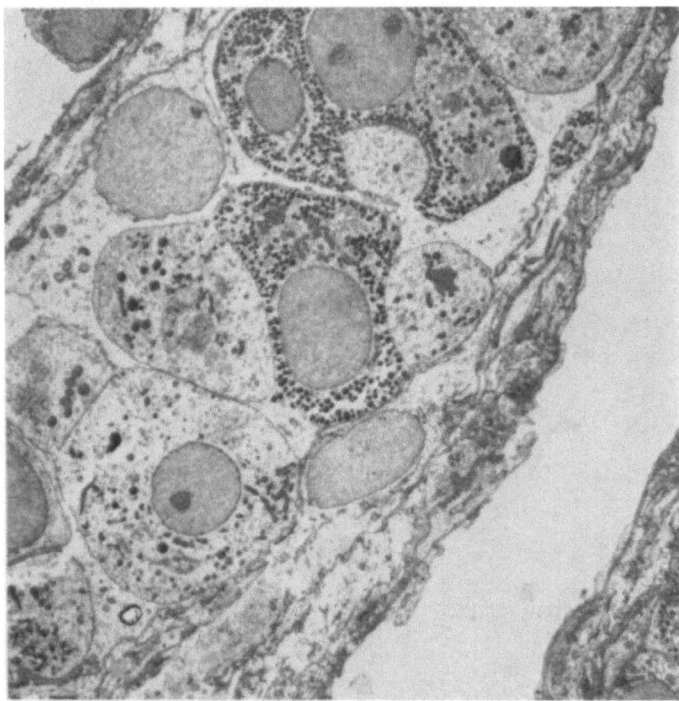

Fig. 2. Normal human pituitary. Lobule of various secretory with different types of granules interposed between two capillaries. Case 36/73, osmium, × 2,400

The majority of the pituitary cells have the same basic structure. The differences encountered are of a quantitative nature involving size and shape of cells, size and configuration of the secretory granules, and configuration of the rough surfaced endoplasmic reticulum (RER) and Golgi apparatus. The parenchymal cells are usually arranged in strands and lobules of moderate dimensions in order that the individual cells never are separated by more than about one or two cells from contact with a capillary or sinusoid (Farquhar, 1961). The individual lobules are surrounded by a basement membrane and a loose network of collagen fibrils (Fig. 2). The secretory cells are arranged densely within the lobules leaving only an occasional intercellular space which is larger than 20 mμ. The nuclei are generally round or oval with only minor indentations and a single large nucleolus (Fig. 3). The cells contain a variable number of secretory granules whose size and structure usually allow the identification of the cell type and the secretory stage. Some cell types contain an elaborate network of RER, one or several Golgi complexes,

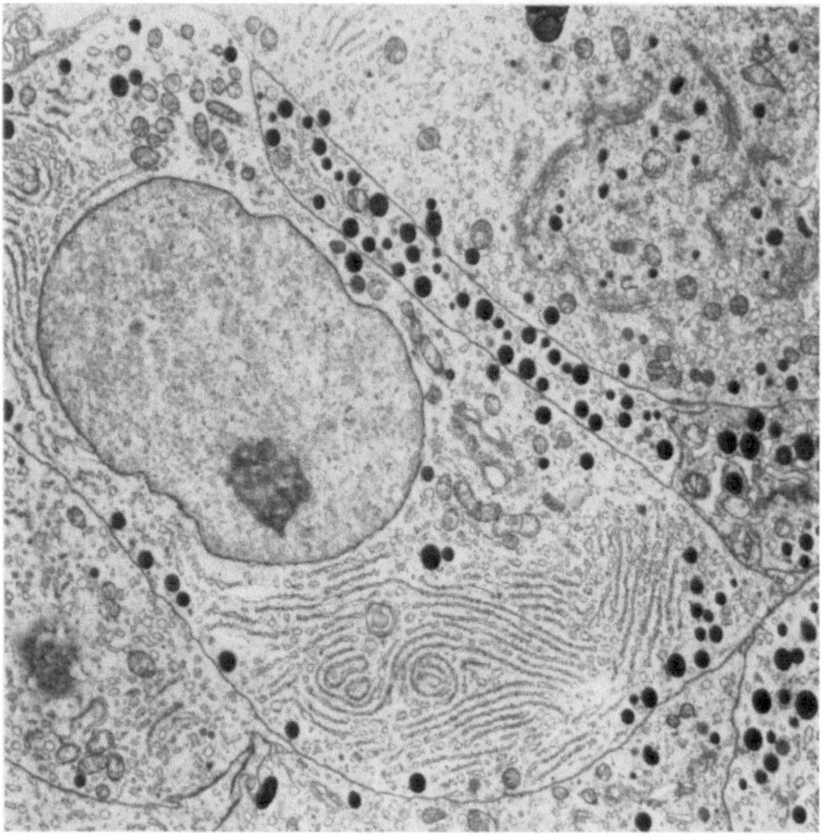

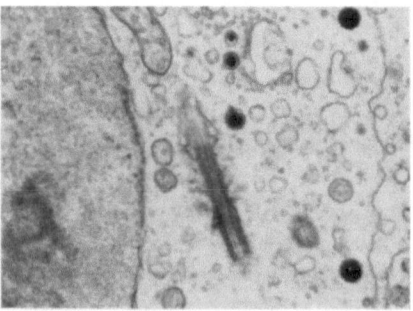

Fig. 3. Somatotrophic cell in normal human pituitary. Large somewhat indented nucleus with single nucleolus, well developed RER, electron dense secretory granules, mitochondria, and Golgi complex. Case 73/72, osmium, × 5,800

Fig. 4. Cilium rootlet in normal pituitary cell. Case 73/72, osmium, × 30,100

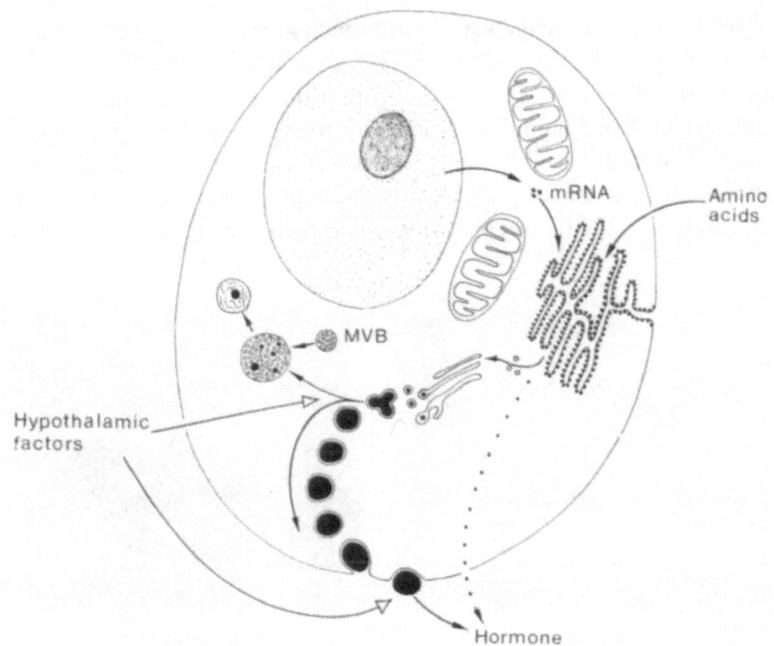

Fig. 5. Diagrammatic representation of secretory process in normal pituitary cell. The hormone is synthesized in the RER under the influence of nuclear information. Small secretory granules arise in the Golgi cisterns, aggregate, and are discharged by exocytosis. The possibility of a direct hormone release from the RER has been suspected. Some hormone granules can be degraded after incorporation into lysosomes

numerous vesicles and mitochondria, and occasional cilia (Fig. 4). The cilia show a 9 + 0 fibril pattern and a two-centriole basal structure (Barnes, 1961). Motile cilia so far described possess a 9 + 2 fibril pattern. Since cilia have been found in beta cells of the developing pancreatic islets from the onset of cellular differentiation, and since undifferentiated, duct and acinar cells do not possess cilia, those of the beta cells must be formed when the cell begins to produce specific granules. The relation of the beta cell cilia to the process of differentiation remains unknown (Munger, 1958). Possible interpretations are: The cilia might be embryologic remnants without a specific function since pancreas and pituitary originate from the embryonic entoderm. They might be chemoreceptors since cilia with the same fibril pattern have been found in photoreceptors (Barnes, 1961).

The secretory process basically is identical in all parenchymal cells of the pituitary (Fig. 5). It has been studied most extensively in the mammotrophs (LTH cells) of the rat (Farquhar, 1971). Mammotrophs from lactating animals with normally nursing young show the usual morphological features associated with active prolactin secretion: a highly developed RER, a large proportion of attached polyribosomes, and a large Golgi complex with many forming secretory granules. The secreted protein hormone is synthesised in the sacs of the RER where it first could be localized with the histoimmunological method by Kawarai and Nakane (1970), whereas the experiments of Tani *et al.* (1969) de-

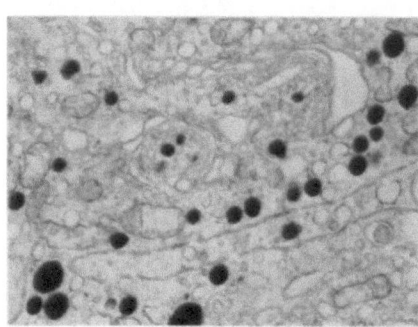 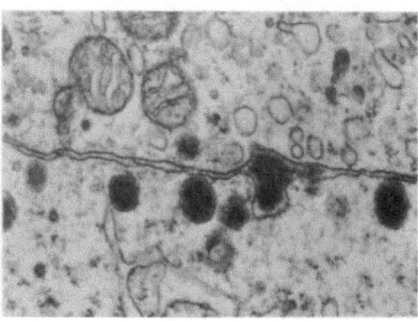

Fig. 6   Fig. 7

Fig. 6. Granule formation in the Golgi complex of a normal human somato-trophic cell. Case 73/72, osmium, × 17,100

Fig. 7. Hormone secretion by exocytosis. Release of granule content into intercellular space by somatotrophic cell.   Case 3/71, osmium, × 29,500

monstrated the appearing immunoreactive material only in the Golgi cisterns. The material is transfered from the RER into the Golgi complex where small (diameter about 100 mμ) lumps of dense material can be detected with the electron microscope (Fig. 6) (Cardell, 1963; Farquhar, 1957, 1961 b, 1971; Farquhar and Wellings, 1957).   This material and its surrounding membrane is subsequently pinched off and comes to lie in the surroundings of the Golgi apparatus. The material seems to fuse into polymorphous immature granules of increasing size moving towards the cell membrane.   The mature granules show a tendency to line up along the cell surface.   This mode of granule formation has been confirmed by radioautographic studies after injection of tritiated leucine (Racadot *et al.*, 1965). The first silver grains appeared after 10 minutes in the region of the RER.   The Golgi complex was marked after 30 minutes. The radioactive secretory granules finally were dispersed among the pre-existing ones.   Some cytochemical evidence has been presented demonstrating that nucleosidediphosphatase may be associated with the concentration and/or discharge of LTH since the reaction product from this enzyme activity could be visualized in the Golgi complex and around forming and discharging granules in the lactating animals. It paralleled the level of the LTH secretion (Smith and Farquhar, 1970).

The control of the discharge of the secretory granules probably is mediated by the hypothalamic releasing and inhibiting factors which are secreted upon action of appropriate stimuli (Debeljuk et al., 1971; De Virgilis et al., 1968; Pelletier et al., 1971a; McCann and Porter, 1969; Shiino et al., 1972, 1973). An exception to this has been observed only in gonadectomized rats after LH-releasing hormone treatment. These animals do not show any granule extrusion in spite of biochemical evidence of intense LH release (Rennels, 1971). Short term cultures of normal pituitaries demonstrated the effect of an acute deficit of the hypothalamic control. The five granulated cell types, except the LTH cells, showed an accumulation of secretory granules resulting in an increased granule autophagy (see below), whereas the cell organelles associated with granule formation remained unchanged. The findings suggest that the absence of the hypothalamic factors may first affect the releasing process of the secretory granules of these cell types, but it may not yet influence the synthesizing process during the short period observed. The accumulated granules have to be destroyed by the lysosomes. In the case of the LTH cell, a depletion of the mature secretory granules and a development of the cell organelles associated with the granule formation was observed. This suggests an enhancement of the hormone discharge and synthesis induced by the absence of the prolactin inhibiting factor (Yamashita, 1972). Pituitary adenomas continued to secrete hormones even in long time culture in absence of hypothalamic factors (Peillon et al., 1972). No signs of granule extrusion could be observed in these cultures. Therefore the question of a possible hormone secretion without granule formation and extrusion remains open.

Each pituitary cell type is influenced by a specific releasing hormone. Neural factors such as dopamine may stimulate the release of the release factors which in turn act on the specific pituitary cells and stimulate the release of the trophic hormone. Schneider and McCann (1970) have reported that dopamine stimulates the release of luteinizing hormone releasing factor (LHRF) from the median eminence. Cyclic variations of catecholamine content in hypothalamic nerve cells during the estrous cycle of the rate have been interpreted as reflecting activity changes of the neurons and related to the anterior pituitary control (Lichtensteiger, 1969).

The discharge of granules occurs by exocytosis (Fig. 7) i.e., by fusion of the granule membrane with that of the cell (Farquhar, 1961b, 1971; Pelletier et al., 1971; Salazar and Peterson, 1964). The content of the discharging granule remains visible for a short time as aggregated lump

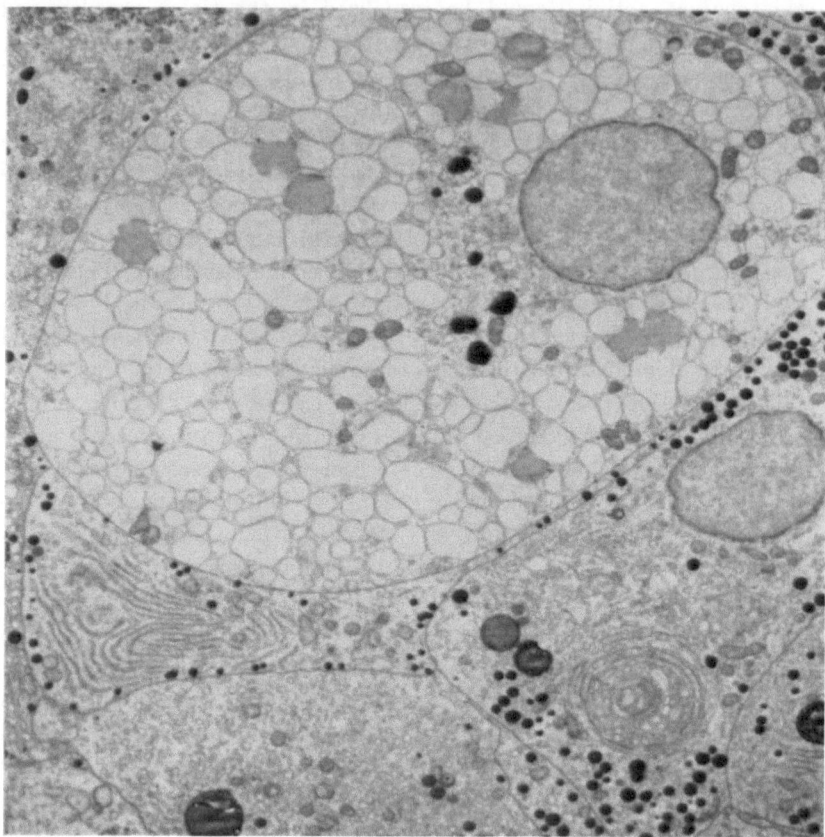

Fig. 8. Ovariectomy cell with ballooned cistern of the RER containing no or only moderately electron dense material, accumulation of numerous vesicles. Unaffected somatotrophic cells in vicinity. Tissue obtained six months after surgical ovarectomy because of metastatic cancer disease. Case 73/72, osmium, × 5,100

of material associated with membrane invagination, then presumably it is solubilized and the hormonal products are free to diffuse to and into the blood vessels. The discharge usually is observed along the wall of the parenchymal cell which is orientated towards the nearest blood vessel. There exists a recirculation of the membrane material used for transport of the secretory material from the Golgi complex to the cell surface (Pelletier, 1973). Fragments of normal pituitary tissue incubated in horseradish peroxidase showed uptake of the enzyme into smooth vesicles which migrated rapidly to the Golgi area. After one hour of incubation the Golgi saccules were seen to contain the peroxidase. This process was not prevented by inhibition of protein synthesis and was enhanced by cyclic AMP.

Extirpation of the target organ (*e.g.* adrenals, gonads, thyroid) results in a chronic stimulation of the related pituitary cells which can be seen easily in the electron microscope (Fig. 8) (Barnes, 1963; Cardell, 1963; Costoff, 1973; Farquhar, 1971; Farquhar and Rinehart, 1954a, 1954b, 1955; Farquhar and Smith, 1957; Foncin and Le Beau, 1966; Kurosumi and Oota, 1966; De Virgilis, 1968; Nakayama *et al.*, 1969; Pelletier and Racadot, 1971; Rennels *et al.*, 1971; Schelin, 1969; Shiino *et al.*, 1973;

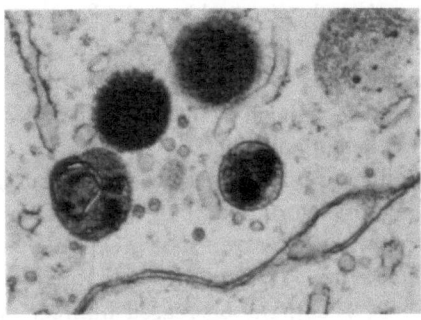

Fig. 9. Lysosomes engaged in intracellular hormone digestion. Uptake of granules into multivesicular body (lower right) and transformation into myelin body (lower left). Case 63/72, osmium, × 23,000

Siperstein and Allison, 1965; Siperstein and Miller, 1970; Stratmann *et al.*, 1972). The cells enlarge because of a ballooning of the cisternae of the RER which become distended with a material of variable but usually moderate density. After about 20 days dense "intracisternal granules" appear within the RER cisternae. Their size and number vary from cell to cell. Parallel to the ballooning of the RER the number of secretory granules in the cytoplasm diminishes. This phenomenon possibly is due to an extremely rapid exocytosis of all newly formed secretory granules. But signs of exocytosis rarely are seen. Since it is known that the specific pituitary cells secrete an abnormal amount of tropic hormones after removal of the target gland (Contopoulos *et al.*, 1958), they must be released from the cell by another mechanism than exocytosis of granules. The mechanism of granule formation in the Golgi complex is probably blocked so that the secretory products accumulate in the cisterns of the RER. The intracisternal granules might be formed because of an increasing condensation of the secretory material. The problem concerning the mechanism by which the hormone is discharged remains to be solved.

After injection of the end organ hormone, granules can be seen forming in the Golgi area. They appear soon in the cytoplasm. The size of the dilated RER cisterns diminishes. Some of the intracisternal granules are taken up by lysosomes (Farquhar, 1971). Sudden suppression of stimulated lactrotroph cells after removal of the suckling young from lactating animals results in incorporation of the accumulated secretory granules into lysosomes (Fig. 9) and successive transformation into membranous residues and lipid bodies. This process is called "crinophagy" (Farquhar, 1971; Smith and Farquhar, 1966.) The process possibly is controlled by hypothalamic factors. Secretory granules occasionally can be found within lysosomes of all secretory cells of normal animals. Hence it has been proposed 1. that in all these cells secretory products are more or less continually directed into the lysosomal system according to fluctuations in secretory activity and 2. that in the secretory cells of the anterior pituitary lysosomes function to regulate the secretory process by providing a mechanism which takes care of overproduction of secretory products (Farquhar, 1969).

The hypothalamus not only controls the acute production and release of the pituitary trophic hormones but also influences the number of individual cell types. The appearance of pregnancy cells (Allanson et al., 1969; Erdheim and Stumme, 1909; Ezrin and Murray, 1963; Hachmeister et al., 1972; Pasteels, 1963), the decreased number of LTH-cells in situ in the presence of an active LTH producing pituitary isograft (Feltkamp, 1970), the regeneration of the pituitary in man (Connolly and Connell, 1958; Landolt, 1973a; Landolt and Siegfried, 1970) and in experimental animals (Cameron, 1952; Daniel and Prichard, 1958; Racadot, 1964), and the appearance of pituitary tumors after thyroidectomy (Racadot and Peillon, 1966; Wegelin, 1925) and after estrogen treatment in certain experimental animals (Giok, 1961; Nelson, 1941; Waelbroeck-van Gaver and Potvlige, 1969; Zondek, 1938) are mediated by hypothalamic factors.

Embryological studies show that the first granulated cells appear in the epithelial sprouts of the pituitary anlage in human embryos of 30 mm crown-rump length (CRL) (about 9 weeks of gestation). Few definite basophil cells can be recognized in this stage with light microscopy. The first eosinophil cells can be observed in embryos of 88 mm CRL (about 14 weeks of gestation) (Romeis, 1940). Electron microscopy allows a further insight into the process of cellular differentiation during human embryogenesis (Dubois, 1967, 1968; Dubois and Dumont, 1965, 1966, 1967). The undifferentiated, embryonal cell is polygonal and contains a relatively large nucleus surrounded by a narrow rim of cytoplasm with few organelles. A plasmodium as described by Romeis (1940) cannot be found. The cell differentiation is initiated by an enlargement of the cytoplasm, development of the RER, increasing number of mitochondria, and appearance of the Golgi complex. The first secretory granules have been found in an embryo of less than 30 mm CRL (7 $\frac{1}{2}$

weeks of gestation) (Dubois, 1968). As development goes on the number of undifferentiated cells decreases and granulated elements become more and more numerous. Three granulated cell types can be recognized: The first type contains numerous, electron dense granules with a diameter of 150 to 600 mμ. Mitochondria are frequent and the Golgi apparatus is well developed. This cell type is considered to represent the storage from of the HGH-cell. Similar granules are present in much smaller number in the cells engaged in active hormone synthesis which are characterized by the presence of numerous cisterns of the RER. The second type shows fewer granules, a prominent RER and Golgi complex. The granules have a diameter of 300–500 mμ and show various electron densities. They correspond to the PAS-positive cells and possibly produce FSH. The third cell type remains unidentified. The narrow cytoplasm contains few organelles and some dense granules with a diameter of 150–200 mμ which are lined up along the plasma membrane. Histochemical studies (Andersen et al., 1970) demonstrate a metabolic pattern which reflects the general metabolic state of the adenohypophysis and which coincides with the differentiation of the cell organelles.

The first paper dealing with the ultrastructure of the adult human adenohypophysis was published by Foster in 1956. This author was mainly interested in the lipid inclusions of the pituitary cells and did not attempt a granule classification. He mentioned that there was no difference in the structure of the Golgi complex in alpha and beta cells. The differing shape of the cisterns was interpreted as an expression of different functional state of the cells. Since then only a limited number of additional papers have been published (Bergland and Torack, 1969a; Deaton and Dugger, 1972; Foncin, 1966, 1971; Foncin and Le Beau, 1964, 1966; Lederis, 1967; Paiz and Hennigar, 1970; Pasteel, 1963; Salazar et al., 1969a; Tani et al., 1969).

The studies have been based on the examination of autopsy material or tissue obtained from hypophysectomies for the treatment of metastatic cancer or diabetic retinopathy. The identification of the different cell types was based usually on the comparison with results of animal experiments or human pituitary tumors with known endocrine function. The only direct identification was done in prolactin producing cells (Pasteels, 1963) with tissue cultures and in somatotropin producing cells with immunohistologic reactions (Tani et al., 1969). The identification of human cell types by comparison with different animal material is rather insecure since it is known that even the tinctorial affinities do not coincide in different species (Van Oordt, 1963). The comparison with human tumor material also is unreliable since pathological cells produce pathological granules which do not characterize sufficiently a certain cell type (see Chapter 4). Simultaneous examination of adjacent "thick" sections

stained with PAS and orange G and ultrathin sections (Paiz and Hennigar, 1970) allows only the differentiation of the classical three cell types.

Table 2 compares the granule sizes listed by various authors. The
values of the well identified LTH and HGH producing cells coincide
exactly. In addition there exists a general agreement that the TSH
producing cells contain small granules ranging between 100–150 mµ in
diameter. The sites of production of the remaining four hormones remain unclear.

The prolactin producing (LTH) cell is encountered only rarely in the
normal human pituitary. Those which are present are underdeveloped
without signs of activity. The prolactin secretion is stimulated by
androgens, estrogens and progesterone. The application of these hormones causes a marked hyperplasia of the erythrosinophilic cells, which can
be noticed on ultrastructural examination as well (De Virgilis and Staudacher, 1971; Pasteels, 1963). The cell shown in Fig. 10 was obtained
from the pituitary of a patient which had received 3 mg of aethinyl
estradiol per day for one month because of metastatic breast cancer
before hypophysectomy. The large cells are filled with numerous electron
dense granules with diameters up to 700 mµ. The granules show often
irregular outlines. The RER, Golgi complex, smooth surfaced vesicles,
and mitochondria usually are confined to small areas because of the
abundance of secretory granules. The cells contain one (rarely two)
round or oval, evenly structured nuclei with prominent nucleoli. The
same type of pleomorphic granulation has been described in pregnancy
cells and estrogen treated male patients (Hachmeister *et al.*, 1972).

The *somatotrophin (HGH) producing cell* is frequently found and can
easily be identified (Figs. 3, 4, 6, 7, 8, and 13). The cell is formed regularly
and is usually polygonal. Their size is slightly larger than the average
pituitary cell. The nucleus is round or oval. The cells are characterized
by the presence of numerous dense granules with a diameter of about
350–500 mµ. The granules are round or slightly oval. The oval shape
might be caused by a compression of the tissue block during sectioning
since of the fact that the long axes of the oval granules are usually parallel. The membrane occasionally can be seen in mature granules. It is
regularly visible in immature granules in the region of the Golgi complex.
The granules are distributed evenly in the cytoplasm. The RER generally
is well developed (Fig. 3). Concentrically arranged circular profiles cause
the picture of the so called "nebenkern" (Schelin, 1962) of light microscopists. The Golgi complex with numerous vesicles and some lysosomes
are regularly seen. The mitochondria often are arranged in clusters and
show a regular pattern of cristae.

The *gonadotrophic cells* secrete two hormones: the follicle stimulating
hormone (FSH) and the interstitial cell stimulating or luteinizing hor-

Table 2. *Ultrastructural Classification of Granule Size in Human Pituitary Cell Types by Different Authors* (Diameter in mμ)

Hormone produced	Bergland and Torack (1969)	Foncin (1966)	Foncin (1971)	Lederis (1966)	Paiz and Hennigar (1970)	Pelletier (1971)	Salazar *et al.* (1969)
LTH	Type 1 500–1000	Type 3 — 700	~ 700	Type 2 300–>700		Type B 400–700	Type 4 400
HGH	Type 2 300–400	Type 1 350–500	350–400	Type 1 300–500	serous cell 350	Type A ~ 300	Type 3 250–400
FSH	Type 3 200–400	Type 4 ~ 500	~ 500	Type 3 ~ 200	β cell 450	Type E	Type 2
LH	Type 4 150–200		~ 250		250–500, 500–1000	200–350	150–200
TSH	Type 5 ~ 100		~ 100	Type 5 ? 100–150		Type F 100–150	Type 1 >150
ACTH	Follicle cell (200–400)	Type 2 90–130	90–130	Type 5 ? 100–150	serous cell 150	Type C 200	
MSH		Type 5 160–200	150–300			Type D 250	
Unknown function				Type 4 ~ 200	Follicular cell	Type G follicular cell	Type 5: degranulated cell Type 6: stellate cell

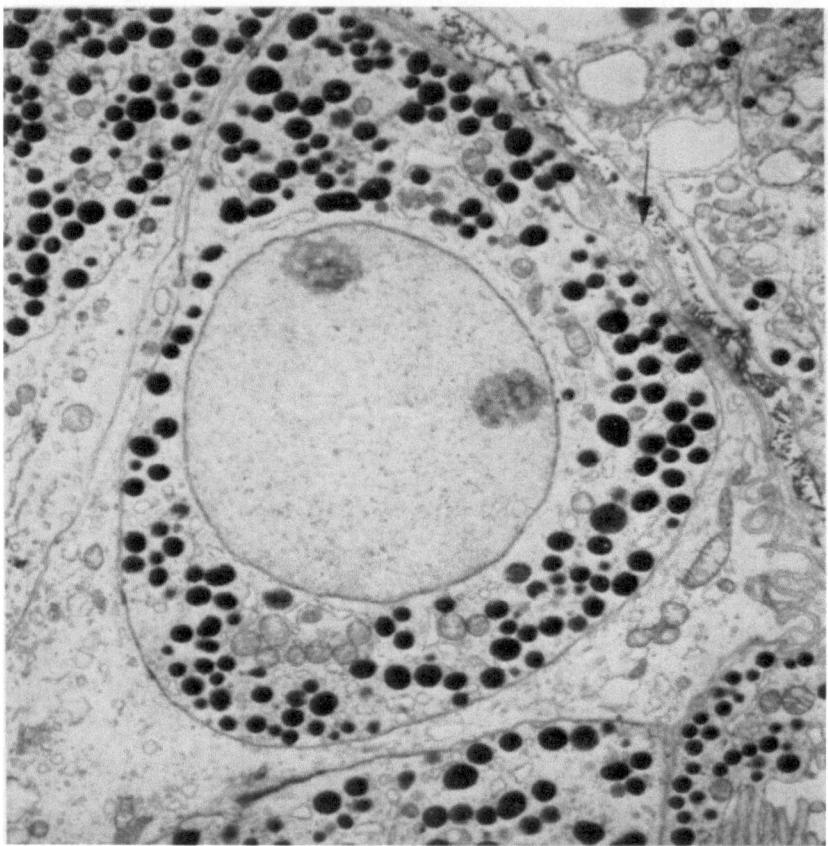

Fig. 10. Prolactin (LTH) producing cell in patient with mammary cancer treated with high doses of estrogens. Accumulation of large, often polymorphic granules. The cell is surrounded by basement membrane (arrow) and by process of agranular follicular cell. Case 73/72, osmium, ×7,200

mone (ICSH or LH). Two different types of cells of the rat pituitary originally were described, each one being responsible for the secretion of one hormone (Barnes, 1963; Costoff, 1973; Debeljuk *et al.*, 1973; Farquhar and Rinehart, 1954a, 1955; Girod and Dubois, 1965; Herlant, 1964; Kurosumi and Oota, 1968). This view was based on the observation of different effects of castration and subsequent treatment with FSH. The appearance of ovariectomy changes was observed within 6 days in the FSH-cells and only after 35 days in LH-cells. The FSH-cells were considered to be larger and the diameter of their granules smaller (150–200 mµ.) The opposite was observed in the smaller LH-cells which contained granules with a diameter of 200–250 mµ. The immunohisto-logic and histologic examination of human pars distalis by Phifer *et al.*

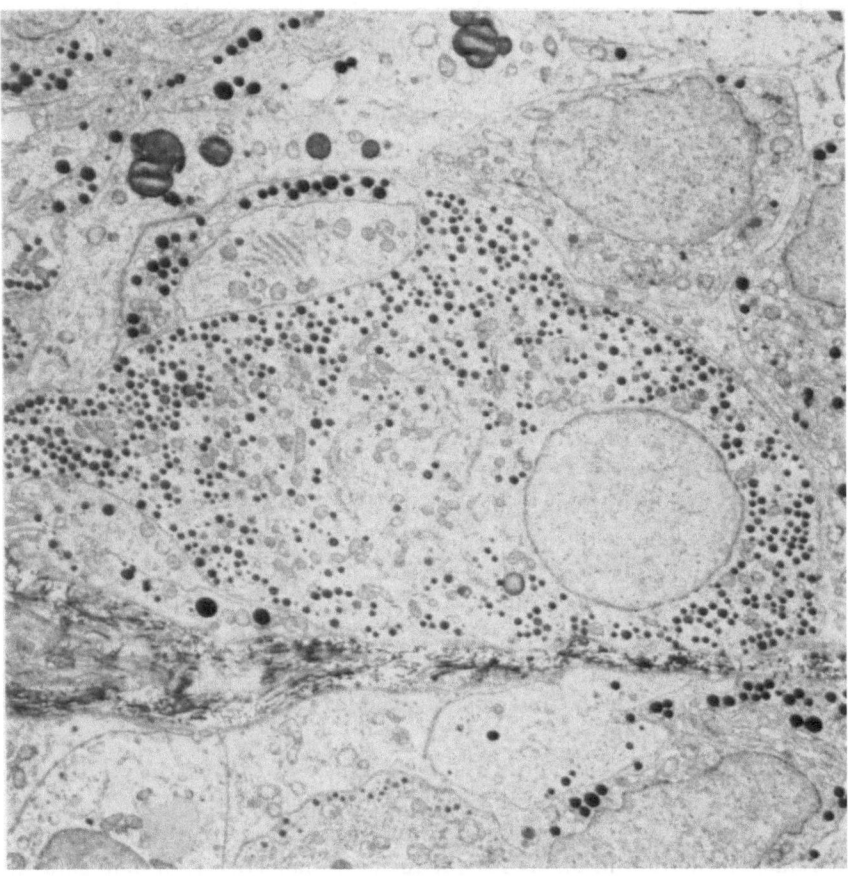

Fig. 11. Large gonadotrophic cell with granules of moderate electron density and relatively small nucleus situated at edge of lobule surrounded by somatotrophic cells and unidentified process with lipid droplets. Case 73/72, osmium, × 6,100

(1973) has shown that both hormones are present in the same cell type. A new staining method revealed that gonadotrophic cells often contained two different granule types at the same time. The immunohistological studies of Nakane (1970) showed two cell types with granules measuring 200–250 mμ in diameter in the rat. The larger cell type reacted with both anti-FSH and anti-LH whereas the smaller cell reacted only with anti-FSH. Nakane concluded that the "one hormone—one cell" theory did not hold for gonadotrophic cells. The different hormone distribution might be only an expression of differing physiologic conditions of the same cell type. Some authors dealing with human pituitary material describe two, others only one, gonadotrophic cell type as shown in Table 2.

The granule sizes indicated show variations between 150 and 1000 mμ. There exists general agreement that the electron density of the granules is low and shows considerable variation (Fig. 11). The granules in our material show a diameter of 150–250 mμ. The cells are usually large and are situated on the periphery of the lobules. Numerous Golgi cisterns can be seen. The RER is sometimes described as not prominent (Paiz and Hennigar, 1970) or as well developed, dilated and filled with finely floccular material (Foncin, 1966, 1971).

Ovariectomy cells (Fig. 8) demonstrated an extremely dilated RER which is filled with the same floccular material showing condensations of medium electron density (Foncin and Le Beau, 1966). The remaining cell organelles are pushed in the background by the vesicular RER. The mitochondria of normal and hyperactive ovariectomy cells are relatively small and dense.

The thyreotrophin (TSH) producing cell contains very small granules with a diameter of only 100–150 mμ (Fig. 12) according to all authors (Table 2). The mitochondria are relatively large as compared to the other cell organelles. The Golgi complex and the RER are scanty. Similar appearing cells could be transformed into thyroidectomy cells in experimental animals. They incorporated labeled thymidine after propylthiouracil (PTU) treatment in an increased rate (Stratmann et al., 1972) and responded with increased granule extrusion to TRF application (Shiino et al., 1973).

The site of production of the *adrenocorticotrophic hormone (ACTH)* first had been localized in the agranular follicular cells (see below) (Farquhar, 1957). This finding was supported by the description of follicle formation in an ACTH-producing tumor (Bergland and Torack, 1969a). Light microscopic, immunohistologic studies later have proven beyond any doubt that follicular cells are not involved in ACTH synthesis in man (Phifer et al., 1970). The changes in pituitary ACTH-producing cells which occur after adrenalectomy support the view that the hormone is produced by granulated and not by agranular cells (Nakayama et al., 1969; Siperstein and Miller, 1970; Moriarty and Halmi, 1972). The ACTH-granule has been described as the smallest with a diameter of 90–130 mμ in man (Foncin and Le Beau, 1964). Other authors have indicated larger values (see Table 2). The granules are characterized by a high electron density and a clear halo separating the granule core and the membrane (Fig. 13). The cells contain nearly no RER. Smooth surfaced vesicles and free ribosomes are numerous. The Golgi complex is well developed.

The melanotrophin (MSH) producing cells can be differenciated from the ACTH cells in light microscopy with differential staining in the normal and abnormal human pituitary (Purves, 1966; Racadot, 1966a;

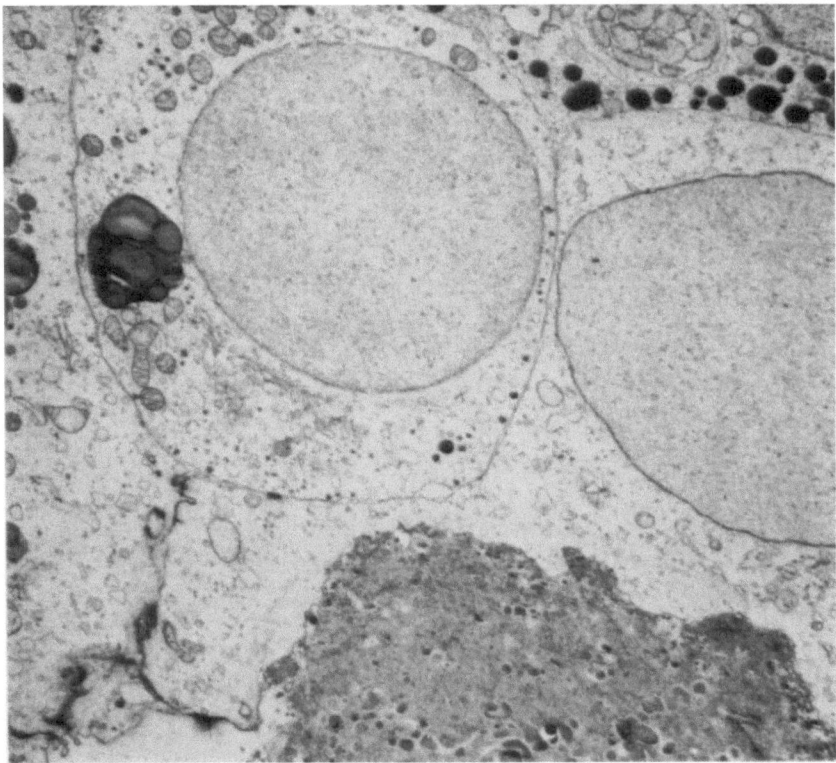

Fig. 12. Thyreotrophin producing cell with extremely small granules and large lipid droplet and part of agranular follicular cell surrounding accumulation of collid substance (lower part of picture). Case 73/72, osmium, × 8,600

Racadot *et al.*, 1966). The ACTH producing cell shows a fine erythrosine-positive granulation. The MSH producing cell demonstrates coarse PAS-positive granules. The ultrastructure of human MSH producing cells has only been described in tumor material (Foncin, 1966, 1971; Pelletier, 1971). The cells have been characterized as polygonal elements with an eccentric nucleus, numerous lipid inclusions, lysosomes, and granules with a diameter of 150–300 mμ.

In addition to the granulated hypophysial cells described there exist nongranulated elements with a distinct morphology that had escaped attention until 1957 when Farquhar described cells that she referred to as *"follicular cells"*. Since then, similar cells have been described in several animal species (Costoff, 1973; Dingemanns, 1970; Dingemanns and Feltkamp, 1972; Dubois and Girod, 1969; Kagayama, 1965; Olivier *et al.*, 1971; Rennels, 1964; Salazar, 1963; Schechter, 1969; Vila-Porcile

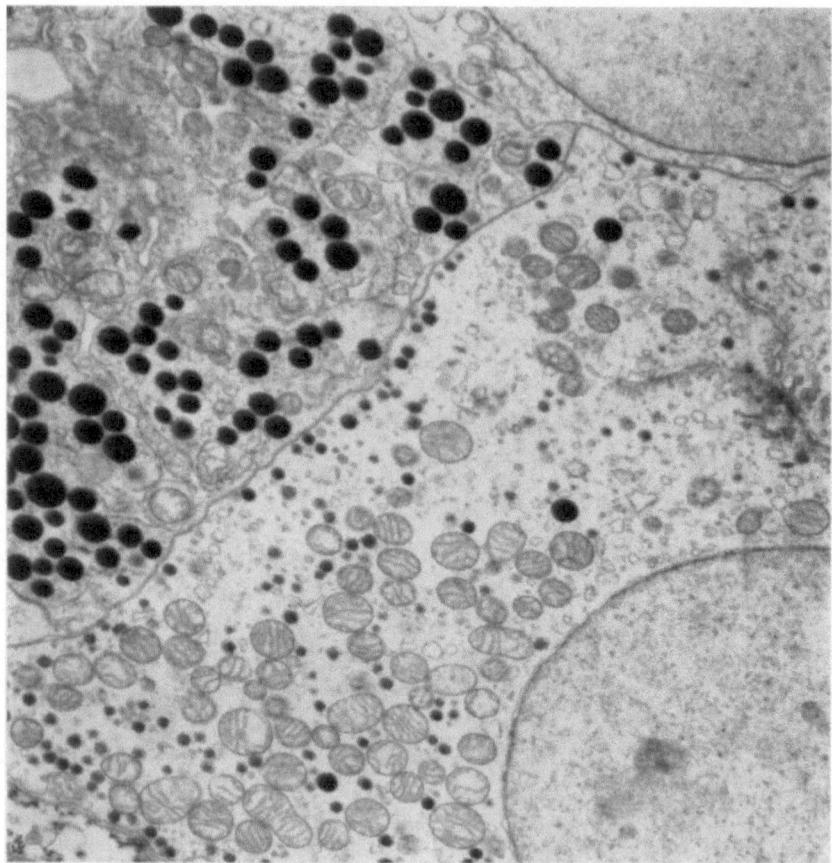

Fig. 13. Part of adrenocorticotrophic cell (lower right) and somatotrophic cell (upper left). The adrenocorticotrophic granules show varying electron density and clear halos between the limiting membrane and the granule core. This halo cannot be seen in the somatotrophic cells at the present magnification. Case 73/72, osmium, × 15,200

and Olivier, 1971) as well as in human fetal and adult pituitaries (Bergland and Torack, 1969a; Foncin, 1971; Fukuda, 1973; Paiz and Hennigar, 1970; Salazar, 1968; Salazar et al., 1969a; Vila-Porcile et al., 1971). Two forms of nongranular cells have been mentioned: one is called a stellate cell, the other, a follicular cell. The stellate cell has a round nucleus which has a similar size as those of the secretory cells. The cytoplasm around the nucleus is scanty and has multiple narrow projections (Fig. 10) penetrating between the secretory cells to which they occasionally are attached by desmosomes. The processes show frequent

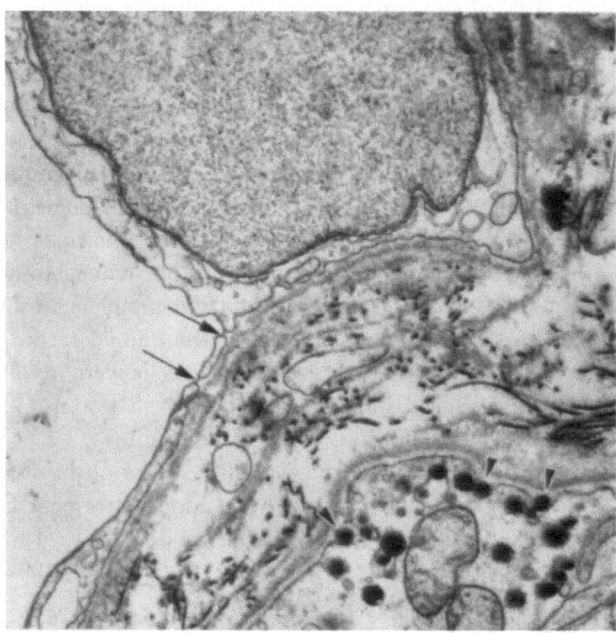

Fig. 14. Capillary and pericapillary space in normal pituitary. Capillary endothelium with fenestrae (arrows) is separated from parenchymal cell showing active granule extrusion (arrowheads) by two basement membranes, interposed collagen fibrils, and pericyte process. Case 73/72, osmium, × 20,100

appositions to the basement membranes surrounding the parenchymal lobuli. No secretory granules can be observed. The cytoplasm contains mitochondria, free ribosomes, and different vesicles. Lysosomes and different lipid bodies can be observed frequently. The follicular cells (Fig. 12) show an irregular shape and delineate small intercellular cavities which are sealed by junctional complexes. The nucleus often is situated in the vicinity of the follicular cavity, but this is not always the case. The follicular cells also show processes branching between the granulated cells as the stellate cells do. The stellate and follicular cells are therefore probably identical. The difference is due to different planes of section. The cytoplasmic contents are also identical. No follicular cells have been found marking contact to more than one follicular cavity. Trypsin digestion of pituitary tissue separates the granulated cells so that they are floating freely whereas the follicular complexes remain intact (Dingemanns, 1970; Dingemanns and Feltkamp, 1972). The follicular surface of the cells is usually irregular, or it may show numerous microvilli. Cilia are observed occasionally.

Farquhar (1957) had proposed that the follicular cells are involved in the ACTH production because of the follicular shrinking observed after adrenalectomy. Cortisone administration caused an enlargement of the follicular colloid masses. ACTH production since has then been localized with immunohistological methods in granulated cells (Moriarty and Halmi, 1972; Nakane, 1970, 1971; Phifer *et al.*, 1970). In addition, Dingemanns and Feltkamp (1972) have shown that morphological changes as those observed by Farquhar (1957) occur after various treatments (castration, adrenalectomy, thyroid inhibition, transplantation) and therefore should be considered as general phenomena accompanying many changes in the physiological state of the animal rather than as a result of the treatment applied. The follicular cells were involved in the digestion of waste material in these experiments. They also are considered to belong to the transport system of the pituitary.

The capillaries (Fig. 14) and sinusoids of the anterior pituitary present the same basic organization as in other endocrine organs (Farquhar, 1961 a; Rinehart and Farquhar, 1955). The endothelial cells are of the fenestrated type (Elfvin, 1965; Friederici, 1968; Rhodin, 1962) showing round areas of extreme cellular attenuation leaving pores with a diameter of 70 mμ closed by a single layered diaphragm with a central dense knob. The perikaryon contains some vesicles, mitochondria, Golgi cisterns, RER saccules, free ribosomes, and occasional Weibel-Palade bodies (Weibel and Palade, 1964), which probably contain a procoagulative substance. The endothelial cells are separated by a continuous basal membrane from the occasionally observed pericytes and the surrounding connective tissue which is reduced in most instances to few collagen fibrils. The parenchymal cell lobules are again surrounded by a second basal membrane. Thus before reaching the blood stream the secretory products originating from the extruded secretory granules have to pass through two basal membranes: a thin sheat of collagenous tissue and an endothelial cell or its fenestra.

No reports concerning the ultrastructure of the *pars tuberalis* of the human hypophysis have yet been published. Ultrastructural and immunohistological examination of bovine and murine material has demonstrated the presence of all cell types of the anterior lobe (Costoff, 1973; Dubois, 1970; Dubois and Cohere, 1970; Stutinski *et al.*, 1964). Colloid containing follicles in the mouse show characteristics which are found in the pars distalis only under experimental conditions. Accordingly, the follicular cells of the pars tuberalis have been considered to be probably in an active state (Dingemanns and Feltkamp, 1972).

We have to rely almost exclusively on material from laboratory animals for the description of the cytology of the pituitary *pars intermedia* since only one paper reporting the findings in two anencephalic, liveborne, female subjects has been published (Salazar, 1969b). Two or three cell types generally are present in the animal pars intermedia (Bargmann et al., 1967; Costoff, 1973; Dingemanns and Feltkamp, 1972; Howe and Maxwell, 1969; Kobayashi, 1964, 1965; Kurosumi et al., 1961; Porte et al., 1971; Stoeckel et al., 1971; Vanha-Perttula and Arstila, 1970; Vincent and Kumar, 1969; Wittkowski, 1967; Ziegler, 1963) of which two are granulated and one not. The first type predominates. The cells are medium sized, rather cuboidal, and have a large round nucleus. The RER and the Golgi cisterns are prominent. The granules are only preserved after glutaraldehyde-osmium fixation. They show a diameter of 200–350 mμ and have a moderate, variable electron density. Pure osmium fixation transforms them into more or less empty vesicles with frequently ruptured walls. This cell type is usually identified as the MSH producing cell. The second granulated cell type is less frequent and displays often a dark cytoplasm. There are only a few electron dense granules present with a diameter of 100–150 mμ. They are often lined up along the cell membrane and are resistant to direct osmium fixation. They correspond well to the ACTH producing elements of the anterior lobe and probably secrete the same hormone. The third cell type usually does not contain granules and occurs either as a stellate cell, as a follicular cell or as a marginal cell forming a continuous lining of the pituitary cleft. The apical surface of these cells is covered by microvilli and occasionally by numerous cilia. The cells contain lysosomes and a number of large vacuoles with material possibly related to the colloid within the cleft lumen.

Numerous nerve endings making synaptic contact with granule containing cells are observed throughout the pars intermedia. The majority contain vesicles with an electron dense core measuring 75 mμ. Less frequently terminals contain dense granules measuring 100 mμ or more. Both also contain small electron-lucent vesicles (diameter 20 to 40 mμ). Endings containing only the latter type are found occasionally. The findings suggest a special mode of hormone release although major differences exist among various species (Bargmann et al., 1967; Howe and Maxwell, 1968; Kurosumi et al., 1961; Stoeckel et al., 1971; Vincent and Kumar, 1969; Wittkowski, 1967; Ziegler, 1963). The occurrence of nerve fibers and terminals in the pars intermedia contrasts sharply to their obvious absence in the anterior lobe.

The follicular structures in the pars intermedia of two anencephalic babies contained two types of secretory cells and one type of agranular, follicular element (Salazar et al., 1969b). The basic structure as well as the two granule sizes reported (150–200 mμ and 300–500 mμ) correspond well to the results obtained from animals. The massive retention of secretory material and the absence of nervous structures may well be due to the developmental alteration of the nervous system in anencephalic subjects. The abundance of secretory products in the cells and follicles may result from the lack of releasing stimuli or absence of inhibitory functions from the hypothalamus.

The entirely different ultrastructure of the *neurohypophysis* has been examined in a wide variety of mammalian species (for review see Diepen, 1962; Green, 1966b; Holmes, 1964; Sloper 1966) and in man. Electron microscope studies of human tissue have dealt with the neurohypophysis itself (Lederis, 1963, 1965, 1967), the pituitary stalk (Bergland and Torack, 1969b), and the infundibulum (Bergland and Torack, 1969c). They have shown that the fine structure of the human material is basically identical to other mammals.

Nerve fibers and their swellings of greatly varying dimensions constitute the bulk of the posterior lobe of the pituitary. Processes of pituicytes of differing length and appearance are seen between the fiber swellings. The pituicytes have large nuclei in relation to the relatively scarce perinuclear cytoplasm. The numerous slender processes contain densely packed, parallel running fibrils. The blood vessels are numerous, irregularly shaped, and surrounded by a system of basal membranes and pericytes. The only other cells seen in the human neural lobe are fibroblasts occurring in the perivascular space. Nerve fibers run in all directions. Thus in a given section longitudinally and obliquely cut nerve fibres can be seen. Swellings occur repeatedly during the course of an individual fiber giving rise to the beaded appearance seen in light microscopy. Elementary granules (diameter 90–200 mμ) with dense cores and "empty" vesicles (diameter 25–60 mμ) can be observed both in fiber swellings and in non-dilated nerve fibers. The vesicles may simply represent "detritus" originating from the secretion of elementary granules by exocytosis (Douglas *et al.*, 1971). Numerous axons contain neurotubules. Acid phosphatase-positive lysosomes can be visualized in nerve endings, pituicytes, and endothelial cells (Whitaker *et al.*, 1970). The lysosomes often show a lamellar or membranous structure. Salt loading, dehydration, and acute bleeding cause the number of granules to decrease and the number of vesicles to increase (Reinhardt *et al.*, 1969; Santolaya *et al.*, 1972). Salt loading in addition causes the appearance of mitoses in pituicytes (Duchen, 1962).

4. Pituitary Adenomas Associated with Signs of Endocrine Activity

4 a) Acromegaly

Acromegaly is the best known of the diseases resulting from pituitary tumors showing clinical signs of endocrine activity. This particular tumor type is found in 29 out of 89 (= 32%) pituitary adenomas in our series. This proportion is approached only by the series of Cushing (1912, 1933) and Tönnis (1953) who reported 28% acromegalic patients. No other series has shown a higher percentage: Bailey (1932), 25%; Grant (1948), 14%; Kernohan and Sayre (1965), 10.7%; Mundinger and Riechert (1967), 12.5%. The exceptionally high percentage in our own material probably is due to two reasons. 1. The author's interest in acromegaly has resulted in an increased number of referrals for this condition. 2. Because of unsatisfactory results of conventional X-ray therapy in acromegaly, every acromegalic patient was operated upon. On the other hand, some patients with pituitary adenoma but lacking signs of endocrine hyperfunction have been treated successfully with radiotherapy alone. Svien and Colby (1967) as well as others have found this to be the case.

General descriptions of the ultrastructure and reports of special features of more than 170 pituitary adenomas in acromegaly have been presented in several papers (Cardell and Knighton, 1966; Foncin, 1971; Gusek, 1962; Hachmeister, 1973; Lewis and van Noorden, 1972; Luse, 1962; Nyström, 1973; Olivier et al., 1965; Peillon et al., 1970, 1972; Poon et al., 1971; Porcile et al., 1964; Racadot et al., 1964; Robert, 1973; Saeger, 1973a, b; Schechter, 1972, 1973a, b; Schelin, 1962; Schochet et al., 1972a; Tani et al., 1969). The typical adenoma associated with acromegaly (Fig. 15) consists of an accumulation of epithelial cells which as a rule do not have any specific architectural arrangement or relationship to each other. Therefore, the adenomas usually belong to the diffuse type of Kernohan and Sayre (1956). The cells vary considerably in size, and there is a fair number of giant nuclei and, not infrequently, multinucleated cells. The intercellular space is usually limited to the 20 mμ distance between the opposed cell membranes which only in rare instances are separated by larger lacunae. Occasional sinusoids and capillaries are surrounded by few collagen fibrils which otherwise are absent characteristically from the tumor tissue. This explains the typical soft consistency of pituitary adenomas which usually can be extirpated by suction alone. In our series only one tumor, which had received X-ray therapy (dosage unknown) 6 years before surgery, contained a considerable amount of diffuse interstitial fibrosis. In this series seven other

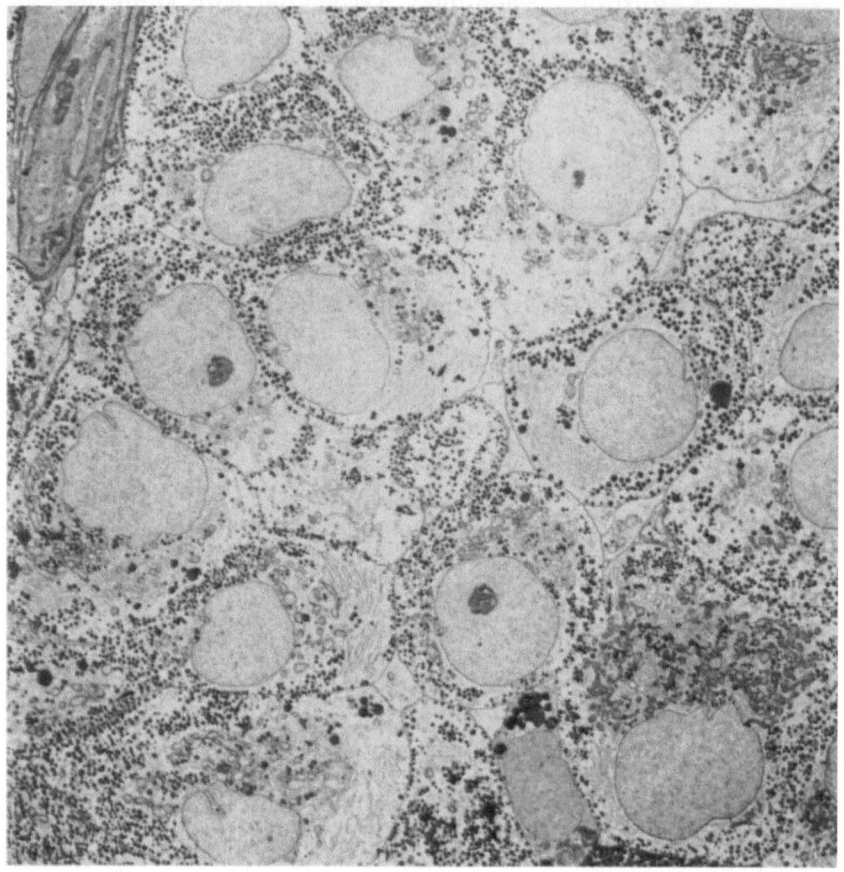

Fig. 15. Acromegaly: Compact accumulation of heavily granulated cells leaving no empty interspace. The cells show large round nuclei, variable amounts of RER, lipid droplets, mitochondria, and secretory granules. Capillary in upper left corner. Case 67/73, osmium, × 2,260

adenomas, which had been irradiated one to twelve years before surgery, did not show an increased amount of collagen. The relation of collagen formation and previous X-ray therapy therefore seems to be at least questionable.

The individual adenoma cell is generally oval or polygonal. Some cells show processes of variable size which occupy the remaining space between the cell bodies. (Fig. 16). The distances between individual cells and the nearest capillary or sinusoid are considerably longer in the adenoma than in the normal pituitary. They reach 10–20 cell diameters. The cells rarely are connected to each other with typical desmosomes.

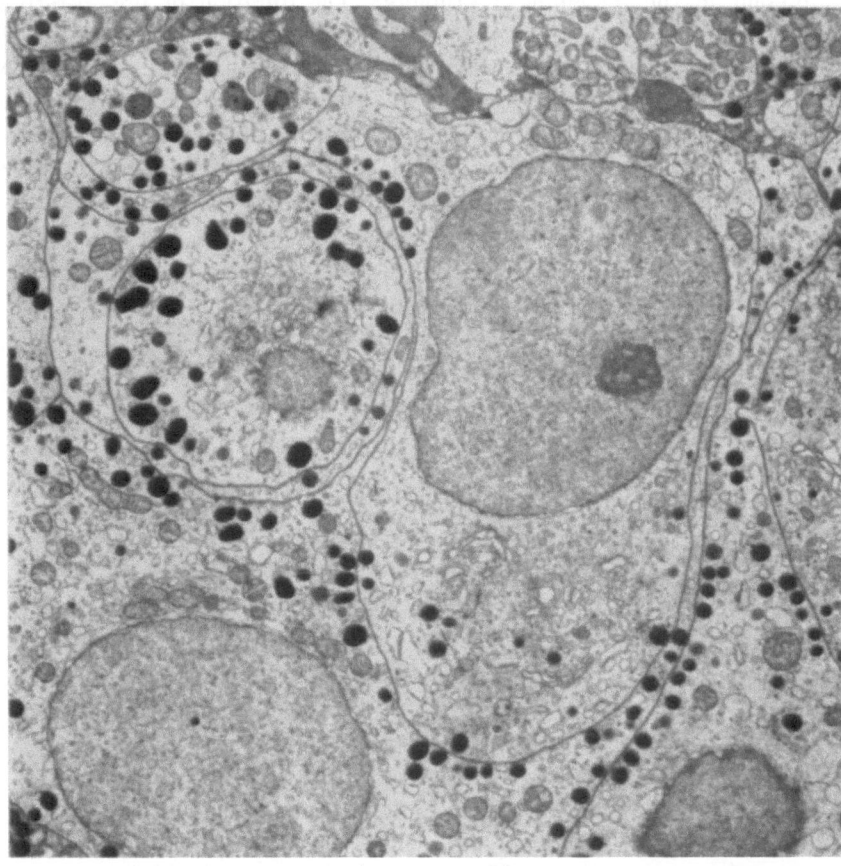

Fig. 16. Acromegaly: Adenoma cells with various processes enclosing other cells. Moderate content of secretory granules which show in this case exceptional polymorphism. Other cell organelles inconspicuous. Case 64/73, osmium, × 6,100

The cells generally have round or elongated nuclei bounded by a typical membrane and a perinuclear cistern. Nuclear pores can be seen readily. The nuclei show occasional indentations of variable depth. The nuclear structure is usually finely granular after osmium fixation. Appropriately sectioned nuclei show a nucleolus. Glutaradehyde-osmium fixation varies the picture considerably. The nuclei show more polymorphic outlines. The chromatin is condensed at the surface forming an irregular, more electron dense edge (Fig. 17). The nuclei of 10 adenomas were definitely polymorphic after osmium fixation with multiple deep indentations unlike the round and oval basic structure present in the remaining 17 tumors.   The duration of pre-operative symptoms was 5.1 years in the monomorphic group and 6.0 years in the polymorphic group with extreme values of 2 and 14 years in both.   The small difference of less than one year is statistically not significant. Recurrent tumors after radiotherapy alone or after surgery plus radiotherapy were somewhat more frequent in the group with polymorphic nuclei (Table 3) although again the difference is statistically not signi-

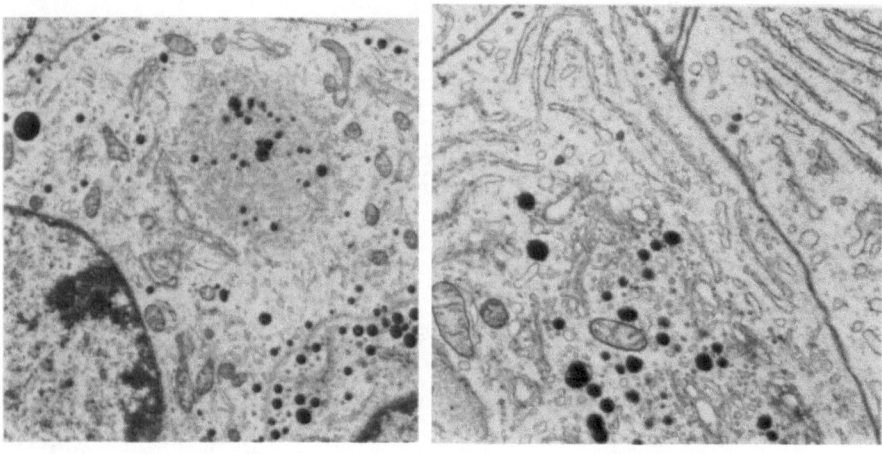

Fig. 17   Fig. 18

Fig. 17. Acromegaly: Irregular condensation of chromatin after glutaraldehyde-osmium fixation beneath nuclear membrane. Round area of filament accumulation enclosing granules of various size in upper center of picture. Case 25/73, glutaraldehyde-osmium, × 6,500

Fig. 18. Acromegaly: Several cisterns of RER and Golgi complex with numerous secretory granules in all stages of formation and maturation. Size of small granules increasing by fusion and apposition.   Case 63/72, osmium, × 13,600

ficant. We cannot decide if this polymorphism is an expression of the previous radiotherapy, if it has no biological meaning at all, or if it is an indication of more aggressive growth as has been assumed for pituitary adenomas without signs of endocrine activity (Luse, 1961, 1962). The results of Brucher et al. (1970) and Lewis and van Noorden (1972), in accordance to our findings, do not lend support to the theory that irregularities of the nuclear structure are sufficient evidence for a more malignant character of the adenoma. Lewis and van Noorden (1972) have proposed that nuclear polymorphism in the context of endocrine activity must be taken to signify secretory function rather than malignancy. Therefore we have checked the pre-operative fasting HGH values in our material. In evaluating the results of the determination it must be taken into account that values above 40 ng/ml serum (normal up to 3 ng/ml) are not quantitated. The average values therefore are to low. Seven adenomas with polymorphic nuclei show an average of 19 ng/ml (with one above 40 ng/ml) whereas 14 adenomas with monomorphic nuclei had an average of 29 ng/ml (five above 40 ng/ml). This result suggests that nuclear polymorphism might be a sign of degeneration

Table 3. *Occurrence of Polymorphic Nuclei in Adenomas with Acromegaly in Relation to Previous Treatment*

Previous treatment	Number of cases with	
	Polymorphic nuclei	Monomorphic nuclei
Radiotherapy	3 ⎫	5 ⎫
Surgery and	} 5	} 7
radiotherapy	2 ⎭	2 ⎭
None	5	12

which possibly is augmented by radiotherapy rather than a sign of increased hormone secretion.

The cytoplasm of the cells contains a variable number of small, round, oval or elongated mitochondria with a fairly regular pattern of cristae and a matrix of medium electron density. The cristae usually are running parallel to the minor axis (Figs. 16 and 17). The mitochondria show oncocytic changes (see Chapter 5 a) in some tumor cells dispersed among the regular cells. The size and distribution of the Golgi apparatus is variable. In some examples there is hardly a Golgi cistern visible whereas others show two or three separate Golgi complexes. The Golgi cisterns usually are located in the vicinity of the nucleus. Electron dense secretory granules and occasional centrioles also can be found in this region. Different stages of developing secretory granules (Fig. 18) often can be found around the saccules. The smallest granules increase their size by gradual apposition of material and by granule fusion. They move away from the Golgi region as soon as they reach maturity. The cisterns of the RER can be distributed through the cytoplasm (Fig. 17) or can form large systems of more or less parallel sacs (Fig. 18). Occasionally circular arrays of the ribosome coated cisterns can be seen which lead to the "nebenkern" formation of light microscopists (Fig. 19). The ribosomes can be scattered free in the cytoplasm or can be fixed in circular formations on the outer surface of the RER cisterns. Small or complex lipid bodies are present in varying numbers in every tumor examined (Figs. 15 and 17).

Sixteen (55%) of the 29 tumors examined show cytoplasmic filaments with a diameter of 10–13 mμ. The interwoven filaments usually form spherical masses which also contain some secretory granules, mitochondria, vesicles and lipid bodies (Figs. 17 and 20). In some instances the

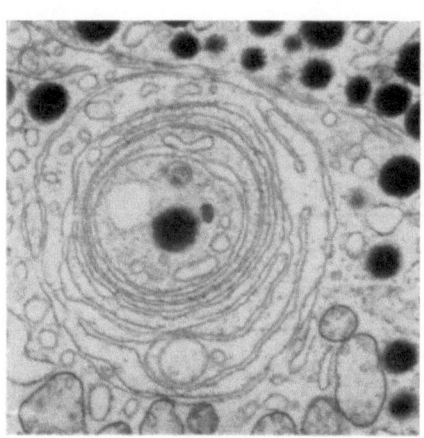 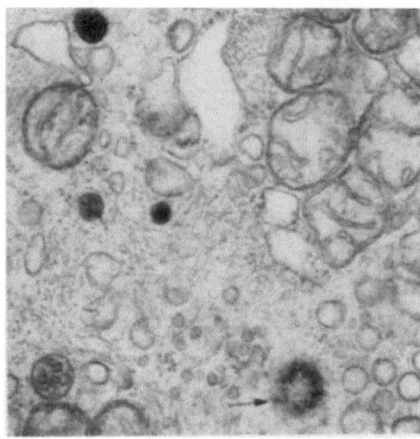

Fig. 19   Fig. 20

Fig. 19. Acromegaly: Circular array of highly developed RER leading to "nebenkern" formation observed by light microscopists. Case 77/72, osmium, × 12,800

Fig. 20. Acromegaly: Detail of intracytoplasmic filament accumulation enclosing secretory granules, mitochondria, multivesicular bodies, vesicles, and centriole (arrow). Case 60/72, osmium, × 27,800

filament bundles are dispersed in the cytoplasm. Similar filaments have been described in pituitary adenomas associated with acromegaly (Cardell and Knighton, 1966; Hachmeister, 1973; Olivier et al., 1965; Peillon et al., 1972; Racadot et al., 1964; Schochet et al., 1972a) and in adenomas without clinical signs of endocrine activity (Oliva et al., 1966; Peillon et al., 1970; Tomiyasu et al., 1973). Cells showing Crooke's changes also contain filaments, but they are arranged in a different manner and therefore will be dealt with in Chapter 4 c. The presence of filaments has been judged as a sign of possible malignancy of the tumor (Racadot et al., 1964) or as a sign of degeneration and regression (Cardell and Knighton, 1966; Oliva et al., 1966, Schochet et al., 1972a). There is no relation between the occurrence of intracytoplasmic filaments and the presence of polymorphic nuclei (Table 4) which also has been suggested as possible sign of degeneration or previous X-ray therapy (Table 5). In spite of the morphological difference between the filaments and the microtubules of adenohypophysial cells, which have a diameter of 28–30 mµ and which have been related to the release of GH and LTH in rat hypophysis in vitro (Labrie *et al.*, 1973), we have checked a possible relation with the HGH level in our patients. Eleven patients with tumors containing filaments showed an average fasting HGH level of 23 ng/ml (with two

Table 4. *Association of Nuclear Polymorphism with Presence of Intracyto-plasmic Filaments*

Number of cases with	Polymorphic nuclei	Monomorphic nuclei
Cytoplasmic filaments	5	11
No filaments	5	8

Table 5. *Relation between Presence of Intracytoplasmic Filaments and Previous Radiotherapy of Acromegaly*

Number of cases with	Filaments present	No filaments
Previous radiotherapy	7	4
No radiotherapy	9	9

patients with values above 40 ng/ml) and ten patients without tumor filaments showed an average of 28 ng/ml (with four patients with levels above 40 ng/ml). This finding does not support the theory of a degenerative nature of the filaments.

The most characteristic and prominent cytoplasmic component are the secretory granules. They are usually round or oval. More polymorphic forms exist among the larger granules (Fig. 16). The granule core is the most electron dense structure of the micrographs. There always exists a distinct, three layered membrane which is separated from the core by a tiny gap. The granule membrane is usually smooth after combined glutaraldehyde-osmium fixation whereas it is undulated after osmium fixation alone (Figs. 21 and 22). A difference in shrinkage caused by the fixation media might be the explanation for these differing appearances. In order to get quantitative data in 5 cases, which have been fixed at the same time with glutaraldehyde-osmium and osmium, we have measured the diameter of 1,000 granules (for method see Chapter 2). The results of the calculated average and standard deviation of each population have been compared in the five cases (Table 6). It can be seen that the resulting sizes are the same in both methods. The differences among the average values are always less than a single standard deviation. The differences can be positive (cases 27/72, 24/72, 34/73) negative (case 71/72) or zero (case 77/72).

Values for the granule size in pituitary adenomas in acromegaly have been presented in several papers (Table 7). Two size ranges have been reported. 1. The larger, more common shows a diameter of 300–500 mμ which corresponds well to the size of the HGH granules in the normal

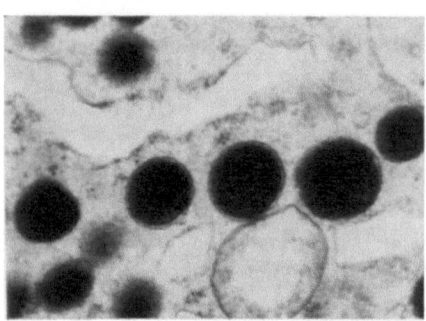 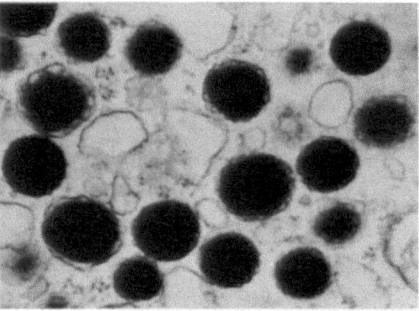

| Fig. 21 | Fig. 22 |

Fig. 21. Acromegaly: Secretory granules after glutaraldehyde-osmium fixation demonstrating smooth limiting membrane with minute perinuclear halo. Case 34/73, glutaraldehyde-osmium, × 31,900

Fig. 22. Acromegaly: Secretory granules of same cases as in Figs. 4–7 after osmium fixation demonstrating undulating membrane with irregular perinuclear halo. Case 34/73, osmium, × 31,900

pituitary (Table 2). The granule size therefore has been used for adenoma classification and identification. 2. The cells of the second type of adenoma which produces acromegaly clinically similar to the first one, contains granules of definitely smaller size (diameter 100–150 mμ). We have examined the granule size distribution in 18 unselected cases; in every case 1,000 granules have been measured. The resulting distribution curves are depicted in Fig. 23a. Several conclusions can be drawn from these results. All cases basically show bell shaped, normal distribution curves which can be described by two values: mean and standard deviation. No asymmetrical distributions as shown by Schelin (1962) have been found. This assumption of a maximum granule size of 350 mμ cannot be verified in our material. The mean values are distributed evenly between 130 and 350 mμ. The two groups of adenomas described in the literature cannot be differentiated in our material which has been numerically evaluated. Adenomas with smaller average values show narrower bell curves and therefore smaller standard deviations than

Table 6. *Comparison of Average Granule Diameter and Standard Deviation in Five Acromegaly Cases in Relation to Fixation Used*

Case no.	Fixation method	
	Osmium average size mμ (standard deviation)	Glutaraldehyde-osmium average size mμ (standard deviation)
27/72	183 (37)	162 (38)
24/72	204 (34)	178 (36)
71/72	265 (65)	314 (57)
77/72	274 (41)	274 (56)
34/73	315 (52)	295 (63)

(Embedding in both groups the same: araldite.)

Table 7. *Granule Size in Pituitary Adenomas with Acromegaly According to Literature*

Author(s)	Average granule size reported (mμ)
Cardell and Knighton, 1966	100–500
Foncin, 1971	2 classes: 120 and 350
Gusek, 1962	300 (range 100–500)
Hachmeister, 1973a	300–400
Lewis and van Noorden, 1972	300–400
Luse, 1961, 1962	300–500
Olivier et al., 1965	300–400
Peillon et al., 1972	2 classes: 150 and 300–500
Pelletier, 1971	500
Porcile et al., 1964	2 classes: 120, 300–500
Racadot et al., 1964	2 classes: 100–125 and 300–400
Robert, 1973	2 classes: 120(–800) and 500(–800)
Schechter, 1973a, b	80–400
Schelin, 1962	2 classes: 150 and 300–500
Schochet et al., 1972a	2 classes: 150 and 300–350

tumors with larger mean values. We have observed that large granules are found predominantly in heavily granulated tumors whereas sparsely granulated tumors contain small granules. Therefore we have divided the 18 mentioned cases with known granule size distribution into three groups according to the density of granules present. This division was done independently by three persons who knew neither the goal of the investigation nor the values of the granule sizes. Afterwards we calculated

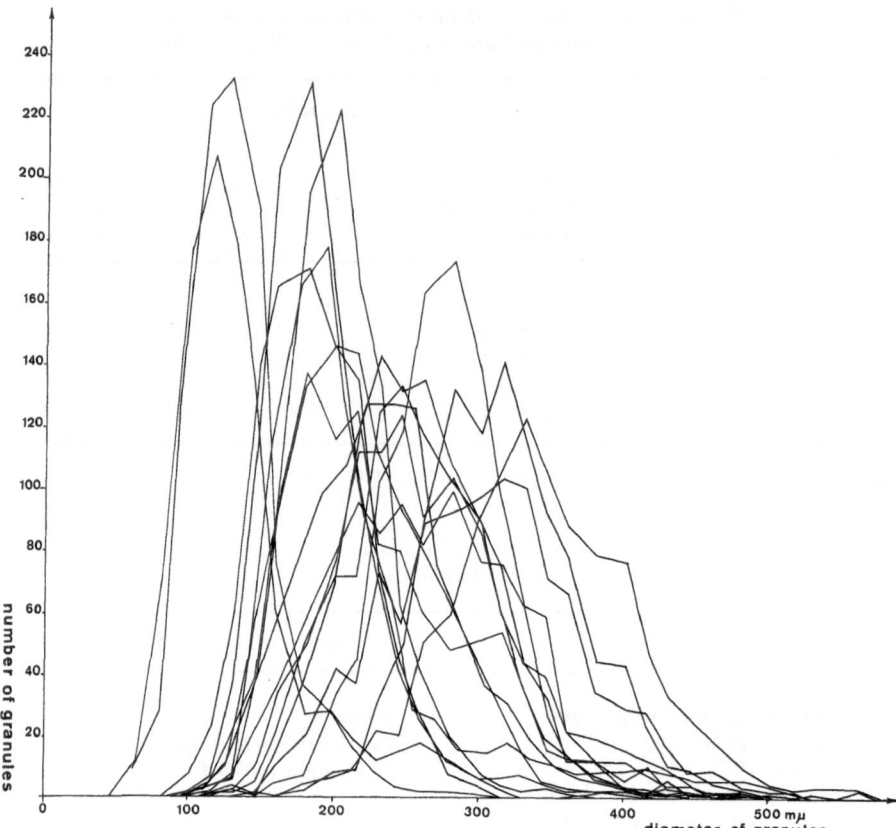

Fig. 23 a. Acromegaly: Granule size distribution curves of 18 unselected cases. For further explanation see text

the average granule size in each group. The sparsely granulated tumors (5 cases) showed an average size of 180 mµ; the intermediate group (6 cases), an average size of 250 mµ; and the heavily granulated tumors (7 cases), an average size of 275 mµ. These observations show that no typical "ripe" HGH granule exists in adenomas. The granules grow continuously until they are extruded. In some adenomas they are set free in an earlier stage than in others in which they tend to accumulate and reach larger sizes because of the continuing growth. The factors which cause all cells of a tumor to behave more or less in the same way are not known. The presence of broader distribution curves in heavily granulated adenomas shows that the hormone production takes place in different phases. The granule size in adenomas is determined by factors different from those in normal pituitary tissue.

Cushing (1912) first pointed out that pituitary adenomas in acrome-

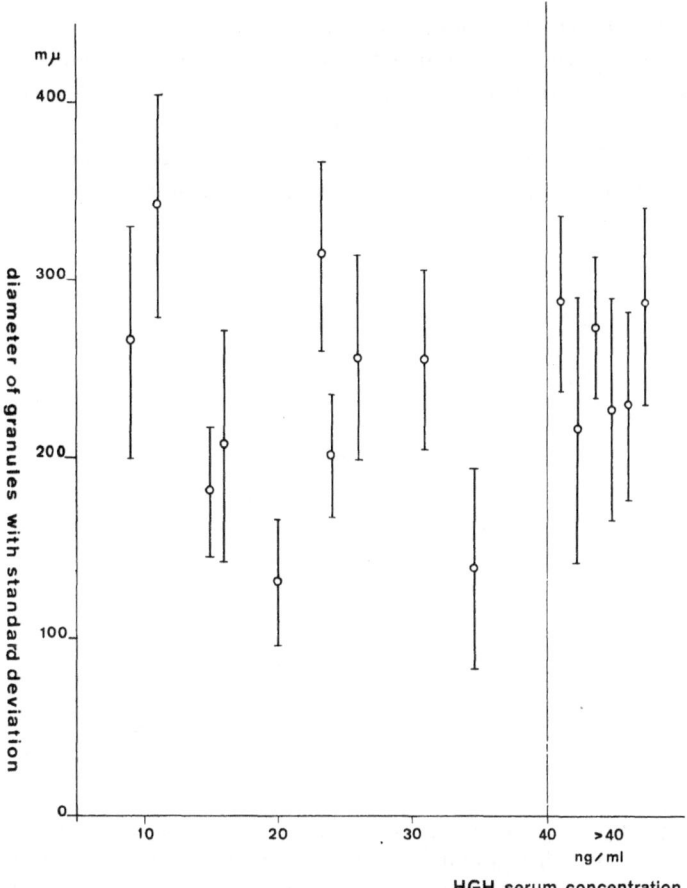

Fig. 23b. Acromegaly: Correlation between granule size (average represented by circle, standard deviation by perpendicular line) and fasting
HGH serum concentration in 16 patients. Cases with HGH values above
40 ng/ml are represented in one group

galy are not necessarily eosinophilic but instead may show the histological
picture of chromophobe tumors. Schelin (1962) using the electron microscope described sparsely granulated and heavily granulated adenomas.
He demonstrated that the staining characteristics in light microscopy
depended only on the content of stored granules and did not give any
indication concerning the secretory condition of the cells. A prominent
Golgi apparatus suggests a high secretory activity in spite of a low granule
content. The relation between staining character and secretory activity
has been examined further by Young et al. (1965). The authors differentiated typical adenomas characterized by well granulated cells, absence

of nuclear polymorphism and mitoses, small tumor size, and absence of invasion into the surrounding tissue from atypical adenomas showing sparsely granulated or agranular cells, polymorphic nuclei, larger size and locally aggressive growth. The HGH content (measured by bioassay) of the individual tumors was much smaller in the atypical group than in the typical ones whereas the clinical activity was much more pronounced

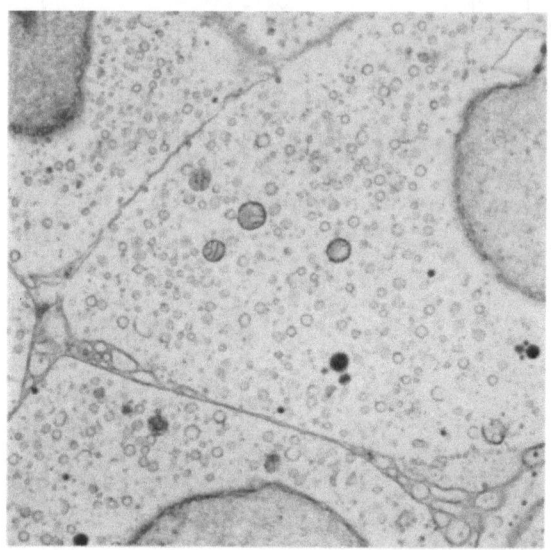

Fig. 24. Acromegaly: Detail of adenoma consisting of cells containing nearly no secretory granules at all. The major part of the cytoplasm is occupied by numerous empty vesicles and some mitochondria. Case 6/73, osmium, × 17,000

in the atypical group. These results were confirmed by the ultrastructural examinations of Robert (1973).

We have seen in our own material, adenomas from severely acromegalic patients containing almost no granules at all (Fig. 24). The major part of the cytoplasm in these cases is occupied by an accumulation of empty vesicles, some mitochondria, and lipid droplets. We have shown above that the secretory granules grow more or less continuosly after the initial formation of the primary granules in the Golgi apparatus. Furthermore it is evident from our observations that the less well granulated adenomas contain smaller granules than the heavily granulated ones. Adenomas with faster granule extrusion causing a high serum HGH level therefore should contain smaller granules than adenomas with lower HGH production rate. We have tested this assumption in Fig. 23 b. The graph shows that no relation exists between granule size and serum HGH level. We have to conclude that the process of active hormone production occurs at a different speed in different adenomas.

Saeger (1973 a, b) has combined several histological and ultrastructural features (nuclear polymorphism, size of Golgi complex, maturity of secretory granules, development of RER) in order to obtain an index

Table 8. *Secretory Activity Index in 21 Adenomas of Acromegalic Patients*

Case number	RER +	Golgi complex +	Secretory granules —	Activity index	Serum HGH (ng/ml)
11/71	+	+++	+	3	> 40
4/72	++	+++	++	3	> 40
15/71	++	++	++	2	> 40
77/72	++	++	++	2	> 40
3/71	++	++	++	2	> 40
7/69	+	+	+++	−1	> 40
64/73	+	+++	++	2	38
29/71	+	++	+	2	35
56/71	+	+++	++	2	31
55/73	+	++	+	2	30
19/71	++	+	+++	0	26
24/72	+	+++	++	2	24
34/73	++	++	+++	1	24
8/72	+++	+++	+	→ 5	20
63/72	+++	++	+	→ 4	16
27/72	+	+	+	1	15
60/72	+	++	+++	0	11
50/72	+	+	+	1	11
25/73	++	+++	++	→ 3	9
71/72	+	++	+++	0	9
58/73	++	+++	++	→ 3	5

+: present.
++: moderate number.
+++: numerous.

of secretory activity of pituitary adenomas in acromegaly. His comparison of the morphological degree of secretory activity with the pre-operative plasma level yielded a high degree of correlation in 9 of 10 cases. We have simplified the system because there is not enough information available to allow one to calculate the final index from the details given. We have graded the average number of secretory granules per cell, the size and number of the Golgi complexes, and the extension of the RER. We divided the individual results into three classes with the following meaning: structure present but rare (+), moderate number or size (++), numerous or large dimension (+++). The number of pluses concerning the RER and Golgi structures which are directly concerned with protein synthesis has been added and the number of pluses concerning the secretory granules has been subtracted. The resulting number is called activity index and is tabulated together with the fasting HGH level in Table 8. The indices reach from — 1 to + 5 and have only a relative and no absolute value. There is a good correlation between the serum HGH level and the activity index in 15 out of 21 cases (no HGH values were available in the remaining 8 cases). Four cases (no. 8/72, 63/72, 25/73, 58/73) had higher activity indices than expected. It is possible that these tumors secrete other proteins in addition to the immunoreactive HGH. Some of the secreted material might be inactive or abnormal proteins or even be other pituitary hormones such as LTH.

This possibility is illustrated by our case no. 63/72. This girl was operated upon three times (in 1960, 1971 and 1972) because of a recurrent pituitary adenoma causing severe visual disturbances. She received a course of X-ray therapy after the first operation in 1960. Each time the histological examination showed a "chromophobe adenoma". The first symptoms of acromegaly appeared in 1971. The HGH determination 7 months after the second operation in 1971 showed a fasting HGH value of 9.2 ng/ml serum with paradoxical reaction during glucose tolerance. This value increased to 16.2 ng/ml 4 months later before the third operation while the acromegaly continued. At the same time she suffered from thyroid and adrenal insufficiency as well as from amenorrhea which was treated by periodic lynestrol-mestranol medication. Galactorrhea started two months after the third operation. We do not think that this tumor acquired new secretory capabilities in the course of time. It is much more likely that there was a slow rise of secretory activity causing the late appearance of the symptoms of acromegaly and galactorrhea. This rise of secretory activity took place in spite of the treatment (surgery, radiotherapy). We suppose that the same tumor cells produce LTH and HGH since only a single cell type can be observed on ultrastructural examination. The combination of acromegaly with galactorrhea is known. Davidoff (1926, 1940) mentions an incidence of 4% in a series of one hundred cases of acromegaly. Krestin (1932) collected eight further cases from the literature. The ultrastructure of another case of a pituitary adenoma secreting HGH and LTH gas been described (Guyda et al., 1973; Robert, 1973). This specimen showed two cell types characterized by different granule size on ultrastructural examination. They were considered to represent somatotrophic and lactotrophic as well as sparsely granulated elements. The sparsely granulated cells were thought to be in an active secretory phase. The possibility of a secretion of the two hormones by one cell type has been proven by cloned cell strains of a rat pituitary tumor showing production between both prolactin and

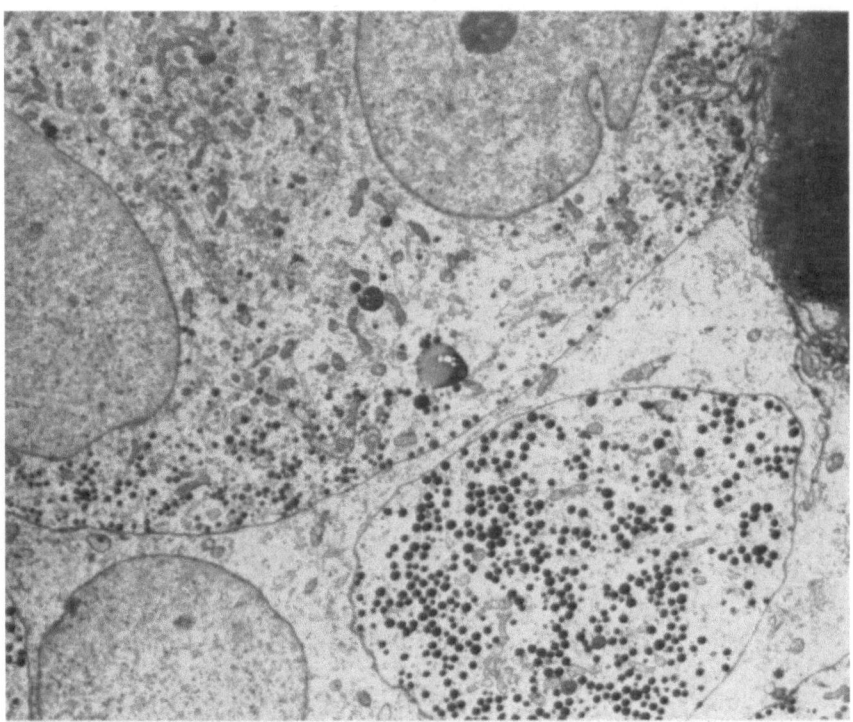

Fig. 25. Acromegaly: Part of agranular follicular cell with stellate processes forming follicle wall around colloid masses. Tight junctions and desmosomes can be seen between cell processes in region of follicle. Case 46/73, osmium, × 3,900

growth hormone (Bancroft and Tashjian, 1970, Tashjian *et al.*, 1970). Stimulation of the cell cultures by hydrocortisone or tissue extracts changed the amount of the relative hormone production in an inverse manner.

We suspect that the negative correlation of a high HGH level and a low activity index in the cases 7/69 and 19/71 of Table 8 might be caused by a stress during the glucose load causing momentary HGH hypersecretion. No other explanation can be offered.

Two specimens in our series of 29 adenomas of acromegalic patients contain follicular cells as a second epithelial cell class beside the secretory elements (Fig. 25). The follicular cells always form a minority. They show a stellate shape and contain only few organelles. The RER is sparse, Golgi are usually absent, and no secretory granules can be found. Some of the processes are connected to each other by desmosomes and form the lining of the follicle which is filled with amorphous material.

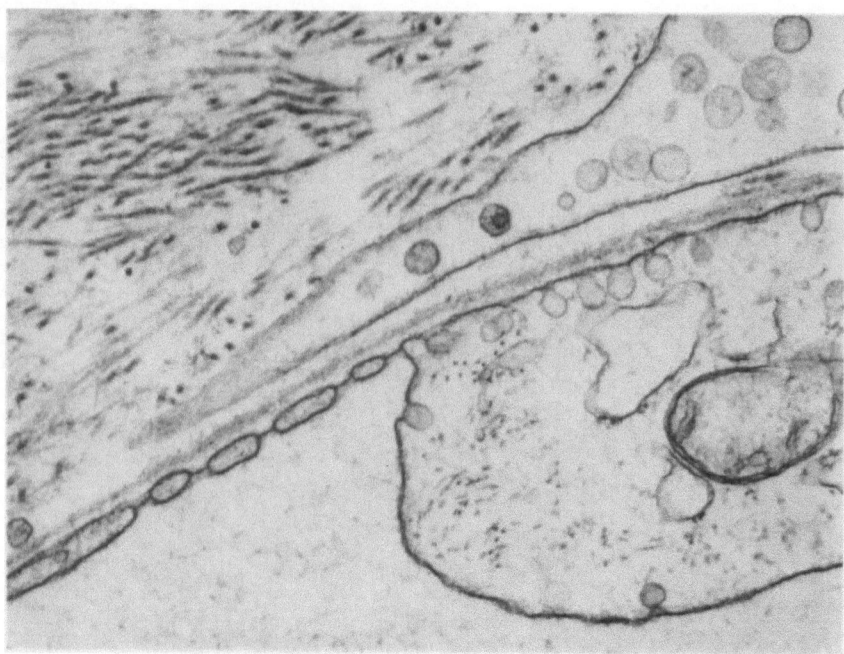

Fig. 26. Acromegaly: Capillary endothelium showing fenestrations and formation of pinocytotic vesicles. Process of adenoma cell containing some vesicular structures is directly apposed to capillary basement membrane and is surrounded by collagenous fibrils. There is no second basement membrane delineating the epithelial component. Case 53/73, osmium, × 46,000

Pituitary tumors contain fewer capillaries and sinusoids than the normal pituitary. The walls of the vessels usually consist of the endothelial cell, a continuous basal membrane, and occasional pericytes. The pericapillary space contains a variable number of collagen fibrils. The parenchymal-pericapillary basal membrane is often ruptured and disorganized (Schechter, 1972). The tumor cells gain direct contact to the basal membrane of the endothelium. Only once we have observed a penetration of a tumor cell process through this barrier. The endothelial cells show fenestrations as well as pinocytotic activity (Fig. 26). They contain mitochondria, some cisterns of the RER, Golgi complexes, numerous vesicles, occasional centrosomes, and frequent Weibel-Palade bodies (Weibel and Palade, 1964) (Fig. 27). Some endothelial cells have a more electron-lucent cytoplasm and appear swollen whereas others are more electron-dense. The nuclei usually are more or less elongated with major and minor indentations.

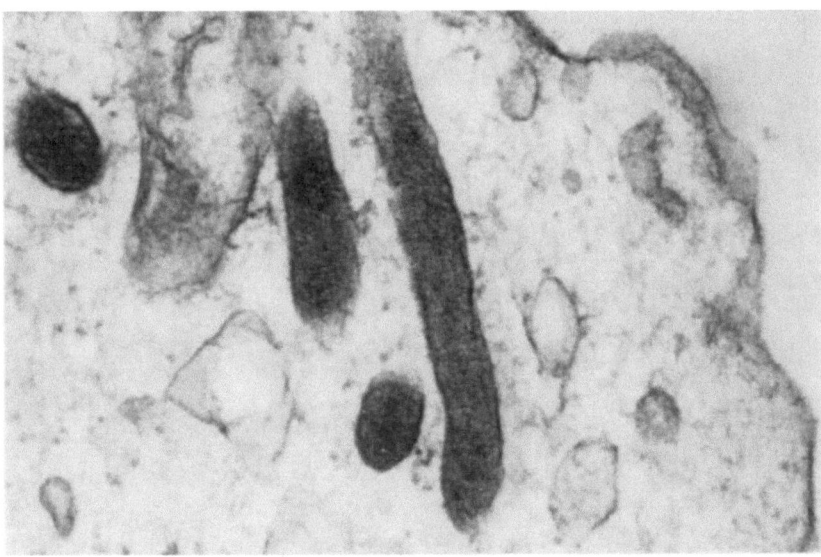

Fig. 27. Acromegaly: Weibel-Palade bodies in cytoplasm of capillary endothelial cell demonstrating internal tubular structure. Case 29/71, osmium, ×70,000

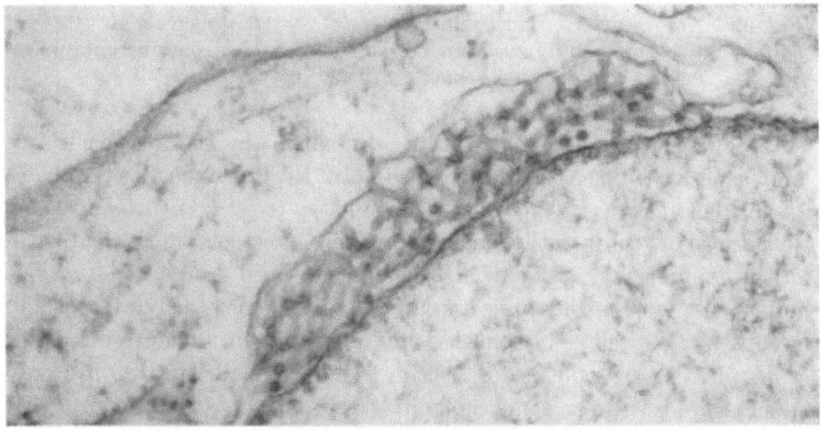

Fig. 28. Acromegaly: Undulating tubular structures in perinuclear cistern of capillary endothelium. Note continuity of tubular walls with outer membrane of cistern. Case 27/72, osmium, ×67,500

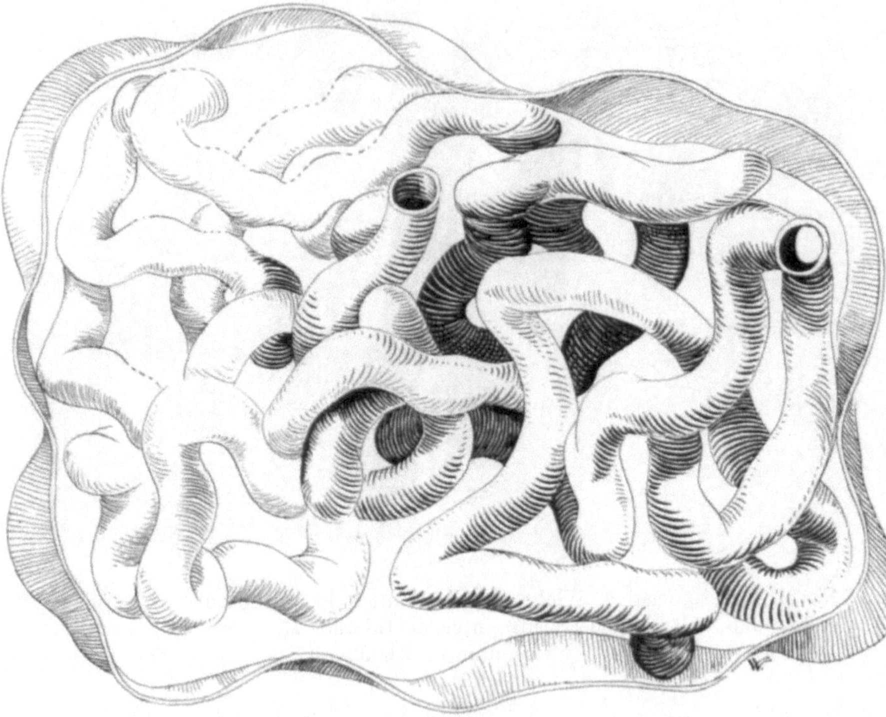

Fig. 29. Acromegaly: Artists impression of three dimensional array of tubular structures obtained from stereoscopy of electron micrographs of "thick sections"

Undulating tubular structures are present in the perinuclear cisterns and sometimes in the cisterns of the RER of the endothelial cells in 8 out of 29 adenomas (= 28%). In some tumors up to 50% of the endothelial cells sectioned through the nuclear region are affected. The percentage in others is much less. Similar structures have been described in various human tumors, auto-immune and rheumatoid diseases, polymyositis and myopathies as well as in nephritis and nephrosis (for review see Landolt et al., 1975). The evidence of their viral nature has been furnished only in subacute sclerosing panencephalitis (Herndon et al., 1968; Jenis et al., 1973; Toga et al., 1969). Similar structures have been found in one case of a TSH producing adenoma (Curé et al., 1972).

The tubular units (Fig. 28) measure approximately 22 mµ in outside diameter and have a light core of about 8 mµ which can be observed only in osmium and glutaraldehyde-osmium fixed material. Stereoscopic electron micrographs of "thick sections" (interference color blue) show that the seemingly branched nature of the structures is caused by the

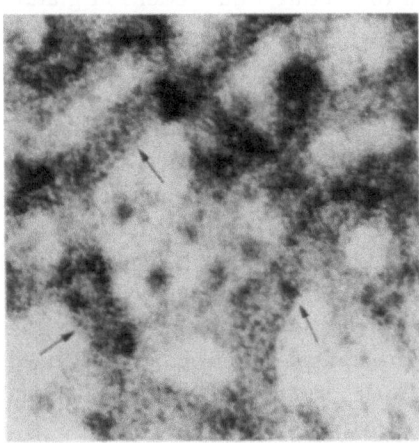 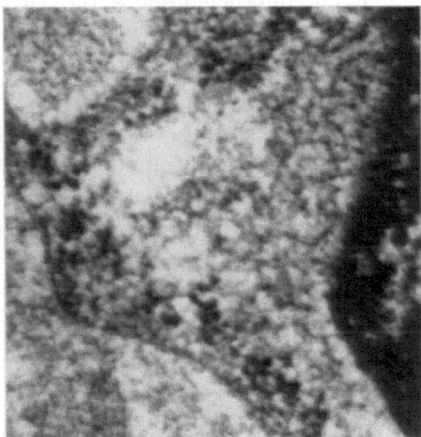

Fig. 30   Fig. 31

Fig. 30. Acromegaly: PTA block staining of osmium fixed material demonstrating cross striation pattern of tubular structures (arrows). Case
27/72, osmium, PTA, × 280,000

Fig. 31. Acromegaly: Demonstration of nucleic acids with glutaraldehyde-
ethidiumbromide in tubular structures showing single strands of dense
material in tubular core. Case 56/72, glutaraldehyde-ethidiumbromide,
× 73,000

superimposition of different twisted tubules running in different levels
and directions (Fig. 29). The tubules appear to be contiguous with the
cistern membrane and the membrane of the nucleus. The tubular wall
demonstrates a unit membrane pattern after any type of osmium fixation. Block staining with phosphotungstic acid reveals a definite cross
striation pattern with a periodicity of 4.0–4.5 mμ (Fig. 30). Omission of
osmium as a fixation agent changes the picture of the tubules completely.
The combination of glutaraldehyde and ethidium bromide, a stain for
nucleic acids used in light and electron microscopy (Le Pecq *et al.*, 1964),
demonstrates an array of electron dense strands with an average diameter of 12.7 mμ (Fig. 31). A definite globular substructure is visible
if viewed in an appropriate position. The unit membrane is not demonstrated with this procedure. Therefore we can conclude that the
strands represent the tubular core seen after osmium fixation. The
method for DNA demonstration with permanganate fixation, incubation
in RNAse, and staining with aqueous uranyl acetate (Yotsuyanagi, 1960;
Yotsuyanagi and Guerrier, 1965) gives a similar result showing electron
dense strands of globular material with a diameter of 8 mμ. No tubular
configuration can be seen in spite of an excellent preservation of the unit
membrane pattern of other organelles. The application of the hydrochlo-

ric acid/methenamine silver reaction to araldite thin sections of glutaraldehyde fixed material results in highly specific silver deposits in DNA
containing structures (Peters and Giese, 1970, 1971). The reaction is also
positive in the region of the tubular arrays in the perinuclear cistern.
The heavy, granular silver deposits in this reaction have the disadvantage
that they cover the underlying structures completely (Landolt et al., 1975).

The tubular structures can be extracted from osmium fixed and
araldite embedded material with perchloric acid. This procedure removes
DNA from ultrathin sections in electron microscopy (Douglas, 1970).
Treatment of p-formaldehyde fixed, 30 μ frozen sections with trypsin
and DNAse removes the structures whereas the combination of trypsin
and RNAse does not change their appearance in the osmium post fixed
and araldite embedded material when examined with the electron
microscope (Landolt et al., 1975).

The results of the histochemical investigations show that the tubular
structures in the perinuclear cistern and in the cisterns of the RER
probably consist of a DNA core coated with a protein layer whose structure differs considerably from the unit membrane pattern in spite of
similar dimensions. The structure might represent a virus-like body.
Several authors (Györkey et al., 1969, 1971; Jenson et al., 1971, Norris
et al., 1972; Norton, 1969; Smith and Northrop, 1971) have proposed a
viral nature for similar structures found in the endothelial cells in systemic lupus erythematosus, nephrosis and various human neoplasms. In the
case of systemic lupus erythematosus a cell-free, self-propagating, cytotoxic agent resembling a myxovirus has been isolated (Moolden et al.,
1973).

The presence of a virus in a tumor does not necessarily imply an
etiologic relationship (Cooper, 1967). The virus may simply be a passen-
ger taking profit from the existing internal milieu which facilitates its
growth. The particles do not have to remain in the pituitary adenoma but
can spread to other capillaries. We have found the tubular structures
in one case in both the pituitary adenoma and muscle capillaries as well.
A further identification of the agent with positive cultures and serological
determinations, which have been unsuccessful until now, will be necessary
for a further insight into the nature of the structures. This will be needed
in order to postulate or deny their oncogenic nature although DNA
viruses are well known for their oncogenic properties (Yohn, 1972). In
addition we have to keep in mind that no presently known DNA viruses
show elongated or tubular structures if viewed with the electron microscope.

4 b) Amenorrhea-Galactorrhea Syndrome (Forbes-Albright)

The syndrome of amenorrhea and galactorrhea with low FSH secretion caused by a pituitary adenoma is usually called the Forbes-Albright syndrome (Forbes et al., 1954) although other cases had been described before (Brown, 1925; Krestin, 1932). The syndrome is rare. Among 430 pituitary adenomas operated upon in the Department of Neurosurgery at the Kantonsspital Zurich in the years 1936–1973 there were only five (= 1.2%) cases. We have been able to obtain biopsies for ultrastructural examination from four of them that were operated upon in the last three years.—The rarity of this particular type of tumor explains why we have been able to find reports of the ultrastructure in only 18 cases. (Foncin, 1971; Hachmeister, 1973a; Hachmeister et al., 1972; Le Beau and Foncin, 1972; Lewis and van Noorden, 1974; Mirouze et al., 1969; Peake et al., 1969; Racadot et al., 1971).

Adenomas causing the amenorrhea-galactorrhea syndrome were originally considered to belong to the "chromophobe" group (Forbes et al., 1954). More specific histologic techniques subsequently have demonstrated that the adenoma cell granulation shows a particular affinity for erythrosine (Herlant et al., 1965; Linquette et al., 1967; Peake et al., 1969), a staining which is typical for the prolactin producing eta cells of the normal pituitary (Herlant, 1960). The biological assay of tumor extracts proved the presence of prolactin (Peake et al., 1969).

The ultrastructural examination of the four adenomas in our material shows that they consist of uniform usually polygonal cells (Fig. 32) containing a round or oval nucleus with a prominent nucleolus. Polymorphic nuclei are only encountered in one specimen. This biopsy was obtained from a patient who was operated upon three times at the age of 28, 30, and 31 years because of an erythrosinophilic pituitary adenoma causing a typical Forbes-Albright syndrome with visual disturbances. The amenorrhea and galactorrhea persisted in spite of surgery and radiotherapy (5,000 rads local dose) after the first operation. Only material from the second and third operation was available for electron microscopic examination. There was evidence of invasive growth in both instances but only the specimen of the third intervention which was extirpated from a dense scar tissue showed nuclear polymorphism. Therefore in this case this was an expression neither of the invasive growth character nor of the radiotherapy given three years before the second operations.

The amount of RER and of Golgi cisterns present in the five specimens examined is generally less pronounced than in cases with acromegaly. But this cannot be used in differential diagnosis because of marked variations in the single case. The number of lysosomes and lipid inclu-

4*

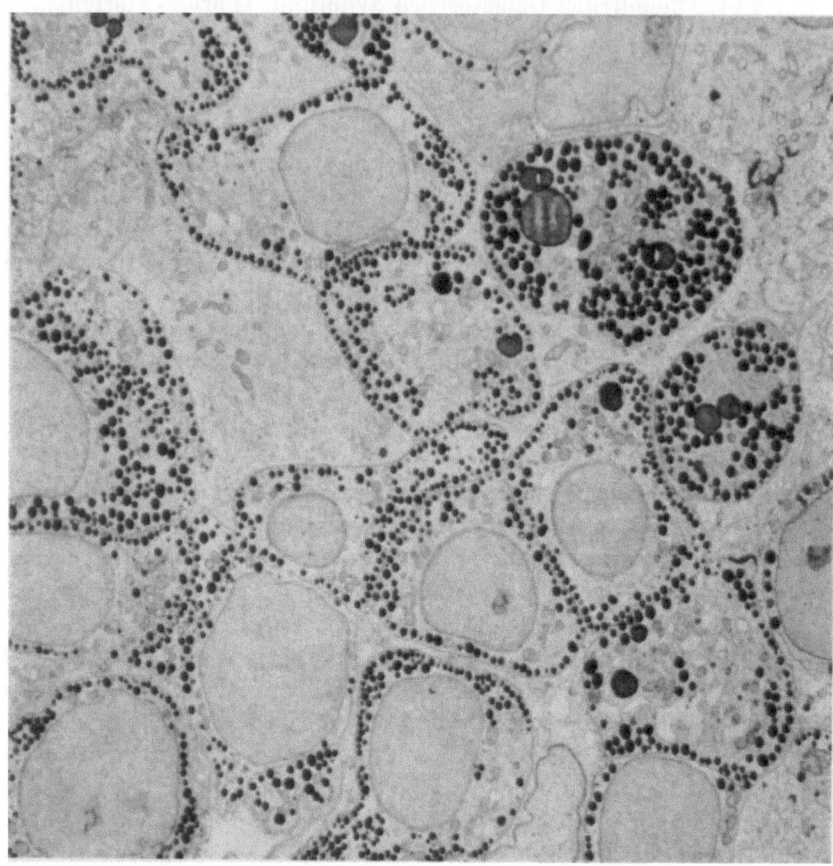

Fig. 32. Forbes-Albright syndrome: Compact accumulation of heavily granulated cells with round nuclei, large lipid bodies, large, often irregular, electron dense, secretory granules. Case 66/72, osmium, × 4,000

sions is greater in the Forbes-Albright cases than in acromegaly. Calcifications were present in the tumor of a 22 year old female suffering for 15 years (age 7 years!) from galactorrhea and primary amenorrhea. The tumor had not been irradiated before surgery.—No accumulations of intracytoplasmic filaments have been encountered in our material nor have there been any descriptions of them in the literature. This difference seems to represent a useful diagnostic criterion since filaments are present in 16 out of 29 cases of acromegaly (Table 4 and 5) and none of 20 cases of Forbes-Albright syndrome (cases collected from the literature and our own material). No tubular structures as described by Hachmeister (1973) are present in our material. This might be due to differences in fixation techniques used.

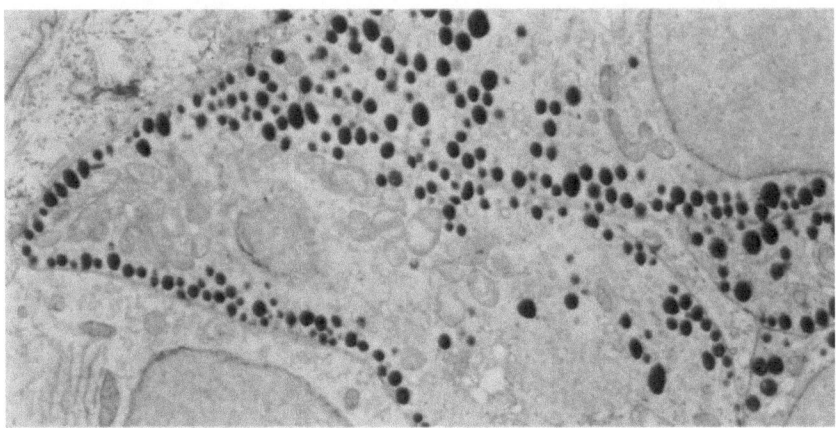

Fig. 33. Forbes-Albright syndrome: Detail of granulated cell demonstrating irregular shape of numerous granules. Case 66/72, osmium, × 8,100

Table 9. *Granule Size in Prolactin Producing Pituitary Tumors According to Literature*

Author	Granule size (mμ)
Foncin, 1971	> 500
Hachmeister *et al.*, 1972	500
Hachmeister, 1973a	400–700
Le Beau and Foncin, 1972	300–700
Lewis and van Noorden, 1974	< 800
Mirouze *et al.*, 1969	90–220, 500
Peake *et al.*, 1969	(200–)500–600(–1000)
Pelletier, 1971	400–700
Racadot *et al.*, 1971	⩾ 500

The secretory granules are the most prominent feature in the Forbes-Albright adenomas as they are in the cases with acromegaly. Their size varies according to the reports found in the literature from 300 to 700 mμ with extremes of 90 and 1,000 mμ (Table 9). The granules usually show maximal electron density and are delineated by a typical unit membrane. Small granules are usually round or oval whereas larger ones have a tendency to be more polymorphic (Fig. 33). One example of our series (case 65/72) shows extremely rare and fine granules (Fig. 34). We do not think that this peculiar picture was caused by a two day long treatment with ergocryptine given two weeks before surgery since this drug causes an accumulation of secretory granules which are ultimately destroyed by lysosomes. The hormone synthesis in the Golgi apparatus seems to remain undisturbed (Ectors *et al.*, 1972).

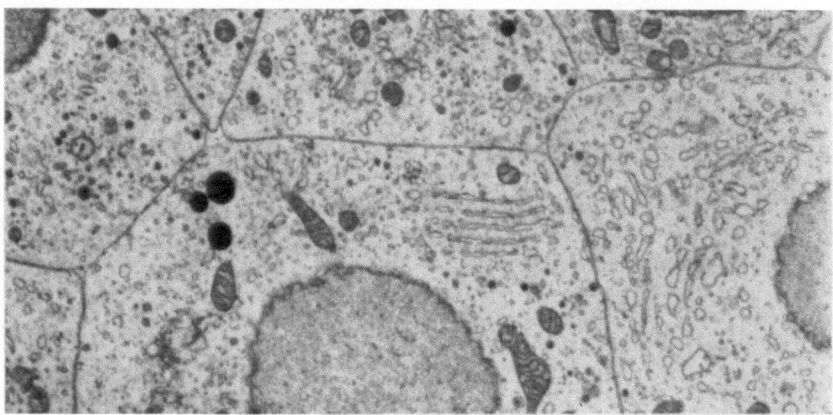

Fig. 34. Forbes-Albright syndrome: Case with very fine and rare secretory granules dispersed in cytoplasm depicted at same magnification as previous case (Fig. 33). Presence of numerous vesicles. Case 65/72, osmium, × 8,100

Table 10. *Secretory Activity Index in Three Adenomas with Forbes-Albright Syndrome*

Case number	RER +	Golgi complex +	Secretory granules —	Activity index	Serum LTH (ng/ml) normal < 25
35/73	+	+ +	+ + +	0	390
65/72	+ + +	+ +	+	4	155
36/73	+	+ +	+ + +	0	25

+ : present.
+ + : moderate number.
+ + + : numerous.

The size distribution of the secretory granules in our five cases is shown in Fig. 35. The average size varies between 157 and 277 mµ (values for acromegaly: 130–350 mµ, see page 38). Only a small percentage of the granules measured show a size of 400–500 mµ which has been judged to be characteristic for adenomas producing the amenorrhea-galactorrhea syndrome.

Comparison of the envelope of all granule size distribution curves from all our cases of acromegaly (shaded area in Fig. 35) with the individual granule size distribution curves from our cases of Forbes-Albright syndrome shows that the granule size cannot be used for differentiation of the two adenoma types as it often has been done.

Blood prolactin levels have been obtained before surgery from three

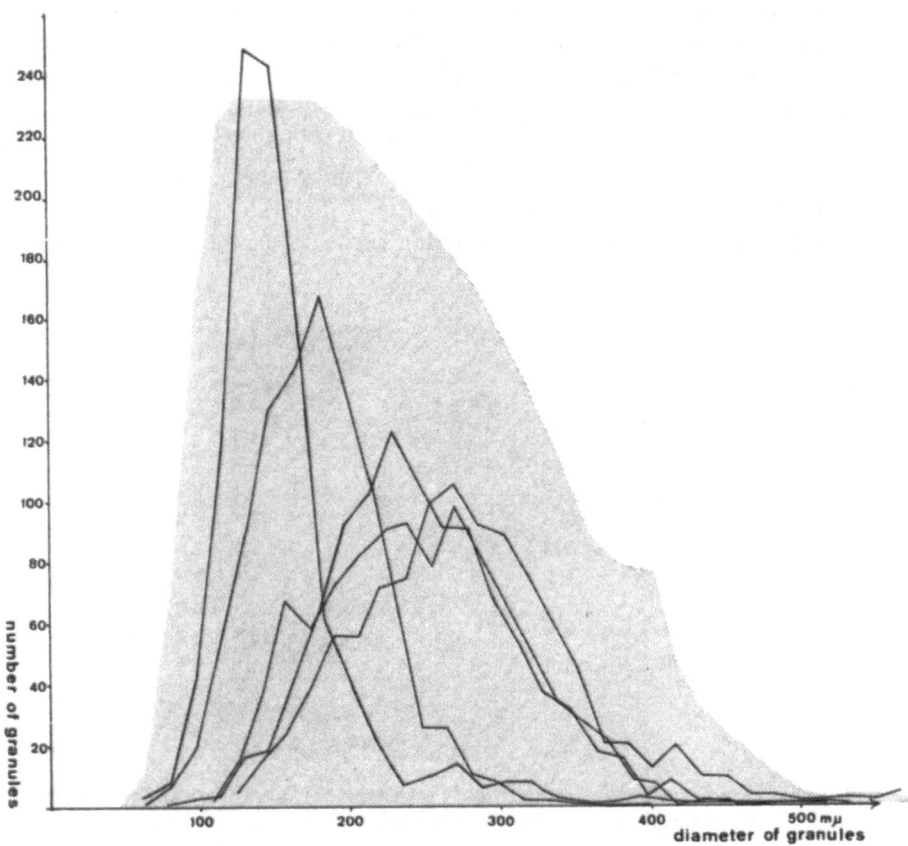

Fig. 35. Forbes-Albright syndrome: Granule size distribution curves of total material compared with 18 cases with acromegaly (shaded area) obtained from Fig. 23 a

patients. They are compared with the secretory activity index obtained from the electron micrographs (Table 10). Case number 65/72 (Fig. 34) shows the combination of a high activity index and a relatively low serum prolactin level as observed in several cases of acromegaly (Table 8). Several fragments of this tumor were cultured. The culture medium contained prolactin (7.5 to > 50 ng/ml) and variable amounts of HGH (0.6–10.0 ng/ml). Immunoreactive insulin could be detected (25 ng/ml) in cultures treated with hypothalamic extracts. This example demonstrates again that pituitary adenomas secrete a variety of protein hormones. There exists also the possibility that various abnormal proteins are secreted. Conventional histology and electron microscopy are not sufficient to determine the exact nature of the secretory type of a pituitary adenoma. A whole battery of immunohistological examinations will be necessary to demonstrate the multitude of secretory products.

Agranular, follicular cells with formation of abortive follicles are present in three biopsies of two patients (Fig. 36) among our four cases. One patient with a recurrent, invasive tumor (case 66/72 and 35/73) demonstrated the presence of follicular cells in both instances. We think that both cell types show neoplastic growth and that the follicular cells are not just persistent normal surrounding tissue. No intermediary forms

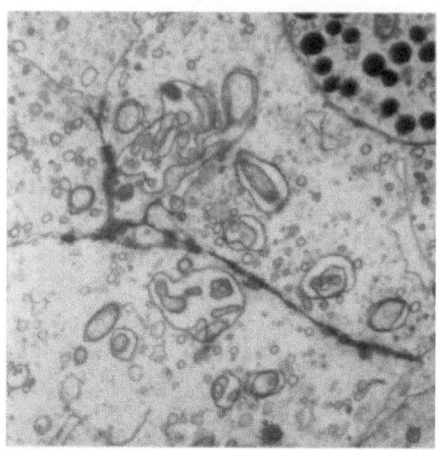

Fig. 36. Forbes-Albright syndrome: Processes of agranular follicle cells forming abortive follicles. Case 36/73, osmium, ×12,200

between granulated cells and follicle cells are present.—The blood vessel structure is inconspicuous in all cases examined. No tubular structures (see page 48) have been detected in the perinuclear cisterns or in the cisterns of the RER. The basal membrane of the capillaries is uninterrupted even in the invasive adenoma.

We have shown above that the granule size cannot be used as a single, simple criterion for differentiation of pituitary adenomas producing acromegaly or the amenorrhea-galactorrhea syndrome. A combination of criteria is needed in order to get some information concerning the correlation with the clinical syndrome present: 1. Accumulations of intracytoplasmic filaments are observed in acromegaly, Cushing's syndrome, and Nelson's syndrome. They are not seen in cases with Forbes-Albright syndrome. 2. The large granules in LTH producing adenomas are more polymorph than in HGH producing tumors. Small granules do not show any differences. 3. Follicular cells and follicle formations are more frequent in patients with Forbes-Albright syndrome than in acromegaly.—

The enumeration of the differences shows that no strict separation of the two syndromes is possible in certain cases. This coincides with the results of biological examinations and with clinical experiences demonstrating the production of more than one hormone by some adenomas.— The simultaneous presence of HGH and LTH has also been demonstrated by immunohistologic techniques in a X-ray induced rat pituitary adenoma (Ito et al., 1972).

4 c) Corticotropic Adenomas of the Pituitary Gland

Corticotropic adenomas are rare. Olivecrona's series of 292 pituitary tumors contained only two examples (Bakay, 1950). In 1932 (a) Cushing described the clinical picture of hypercorticism. He suggested that the characteristic syndrome of obesity, plethora, osteoporosis, hypertension, purple striae of the trunk, and hirsutism was the result of a basophilic adenoma of the pituitary gland. Many of the pathologically confirmed cases published in the following years did in fact have basophilic tumors of the hypophysis which were often of minute dimensions (Plotz et al., 1952). However, equally large numbers of cases were found to suffer from tumorous adrenal glands. Four different etiologies of the Cushing's syndrome have been described (Marks, 1959; Montgomery, 1964; Plotz et al., 1952; Welbourn et al., 1971). 1. It may be due to excessive steroid secretion by an autonomous adrenal adenoma or carcinoma. 2. In others it develops in association with a malignant tumor elsewhere, e.g. lungs, thymus, ovary, pancreas as a paraneoplastic syndrome. 3. In a smaller proportion (10–25%) it appears to be secondary to a pituitary tumor. 4. In the majority (about 50% of the cases) in which adrenal hyperplasia is a feature, the etiology is not established, but the possibility of a pituitary micro-adenoma which does not cause raiological changes of the sella structure usually is not excluded.

A large number of light microscopic studies have described basophilic, mixed basophilic-chromophobe, chromophobe and even eosinophilic adenomas in patients with Cushing's syndrome. Table 11 shows that there is great variation in the frequency of the different staining characteristics. The high percentage of malignant (with distant metastases) and locally invasive tumors in this disease when compared with other pituitary tumor syndromes is particularly noteworthy (Lindholm et al., 1969, Marks, 1959).

Nelson and collaborators (1958) described a syndrome characterized by the appearance of a pituitary tumor producing large quantities of MSH with extensive skin pigmentation noticed some years after bilateral adrenalectomy for the treatment of Cushing's syndrome. A number of additional observations have been reported more recently (Montgomery

Table 11. *Histological Characteristics in 3 Series of Pituitary Tumors Associated with Cushing's Syndrome*

Histological findings, staining characteristic	Marks, 1959	Montgomery, 1964	Plotz *et al.*, 1952
Basophilic	2	4	24
Mixed basophilic-chromophobe	2	3	3
Chromophobe	15	23	5
Eosinophilic		1	1
Choristoma of posterior lobe		1	
Invasive tumor	5		
Metastasizing tumor	4	5	1

et al., 1959; Nelson and Sprunt, 1964). Pituitary adenomas of this type show no stainable granules and are therefore classified as chromophobe. These adenomas usually are interpreted as pre-existing in a micro-adenoma stage subsequent to adrenalectomy. Their growth is stimulated by the surgical removal of the hyperplastic adrenals (Marks, 1959; Racadot *et al.*, 1966a) although differing views have been proposed suggesting a reactive origin of the piuitary neoplasm (Nelson *et al.*, 1958; Rees and Bayliss, 1959).

Romeis (1940) was not yet able to localize the production sites of ACTH and MSH in different cell types. Subsequent histological investigations (for review see Purves, 1966) have been able to differentiate two cell types with different staining characteristics, each one responsible for the synthesis of a single hormone. Racadot and collaborators (1966a) have proposed that Cushing's syndrome can be produced either by corticotropic or melanotropic adenomas. This is easily understandable since both hormone molecules share a long sequence of amino acids. The ACTH and β-MSH molecule contain corticotropic as well as melanotropic activities in differing proportions (Evans *et al.*, 1966).—A variety of the usual Cushing's syndrome additionally characterized by an excessive skin pigmentation has been described (De Gennes *et al.*, 1963; Rees and Bayliss, 1959; Salassa *et al.*, 1959) demonstrating that at least some of the pituitary adenomas are able to secrete both principles. Bahn and collaborators (1960) have reported the presence of melanocyte-stimulating and adrenocorticotropic activities with the help of biological assays in a number of pituitary adenomas from patients with Cushing's syndrome. The simulataneous production of ACTH and MSH by a single cloned pituitary cell line has been demonstrated by bio-assay and radio-immunoassay (Orth *et al.*, 1973).

The further histological investigation of chromophobe adenomas responsible for Cushing's syndrome with Herlant's tetrachrome stain (Herlant, 1960) demonstrated the presence of fine erythrosinophilic granules (Herlant and Decourt, 1964).—This cell type has been identified as an ACTH producing element. A dense granule accumulation can occasionally cause an acidophil staining characteristic whereas a loss of granules due to increased secretory activity produces "chromophobe" cells (Bricaire *et al.*, 1973; Racadot, 1966b; Racadot *et al.*, 1966a).

The basophilic cells observed in the third adenoma type demonstrate the staining characteristics that have been related to the melanotropic cells (Purves and Basset, 1963). The bsophilic cells of the intermediate lobe in animals containing a pituitary cleft are dispersed in the anterior lobe and invade the posterior lobe in adult man who loses the pituitary cleft during ontogenesis. The same cell type is transformed into Crooke cells (Crooke, 1935) or shows up in the initial phase of transformation to PAS-positive hyalin (Schochet *et al.*, 1972b) in the course of hypercorticism of external (steroid medication) or internal (Cushing's syndrome of various origin) cause (Bricaire *et al.*, 1973; Ezrin and Murray, 1963; Gilbert-Dreyfuss and Zara, 1951; Golden *et al.*, 1950; Halmi *et al.*, 1971; Kepeler, 1945; Kilby *et al.*, 1957; Laqueur, 1950; Montandon, 1957; Racadot, 1966b; Racadot *et al.*, 1966a, 1970). The severity of Crooke's hyalinization is dependent on the duration of glucocorticoid administration. The first changes can be seen 72 hours after onset of the medication. Discontinuation of therapy for two or more days decreases the cellular changes (Halmi *et al.*, 1971; Montandon, 1957; Kilby *et al.*, 1957).

The ultrastructure of Crooke's cells has been reported in the normal pituitary tissue surrounding an adenoma causing a Cushing's syndrome (Wågermark and Wersäll, 1968), the pituitary in Cushing's disease (Porcile and Racadot, 1966; Saeger, 1973c), and several cases (autopsy material) which had been treated for a various length of time with steroids because of neoplastic discase, lupus erythematosus, polymyositis, and liver cirrhosis (De Cicco *et al.*, 1972; Hachmeister *et al.*, 1971). The ultrastructural findings basically were identical in spite of variations in intensity (from cell to cell and from case to case) present in patients with exogenous induction. The hyaline zone seen by light microscopy in the rather large cells (20 μ) consisted on the ultrastructural level of an accumulation of filaments. The filaments measured 7 mμ in diameter, lacked a periodicity and occurred in bundles of varying dimensions which usually were arranged in circular fashion near the periphery of the cell so as to enclose the other cell organelles near the nucleus. A minor portion of organelles was trapped between the filament zone and the cell membrane. Cells in a less advanced stage of hyalinization showed filament bundles running in different directions between granules and other organelles which had not yet been displaced. The granules had diameters of 350–450 mμ (Wågermark and Wersäll, 1968), 330 mμ (Porcile and Racadot, 1966) or 300–400 mμ (De Cicco et al., 1972) in spite of their different neoplastic and reactive origins. Their electron density showed variations. Usually cells also contained large lipid inclusions and lysosomes.—The presence of small bundles of filaments measuring 6–8 mμ in diameter also has been used for identification of beta 1 basophils in patients with Hurler's syndrome who had not received any previous steroid medication (Schochet et al., 1974).

Basically two types of pituitary adenomas causing Cushing's syndrome have been reported in the literature. One of them contained Crooke cells, the other did not. We have been able to collect a total of 27 cases from seven papers (Table 12). This number of cases is probably somewhat too high since some cases may have been reported more than once. The distribution of granule sizes in these two types of adenomas can be seen in Table 12. The cases with Crooke cells seem to contain larger granules than those without Crooke cells. The latter have granules which most often are situated in the region of the Golgi cisterns and lined up along the cell membrane. Three granule classes have been described by Olivier and collaborators (1972). Each class usually formed the majority of the granule population of one cell type. The three resulting cell types often were mixed in a single tumor. In some cases there existed one predominating cell type and rarely was the only one present. Immunohistologic examinations demonstrated the presence of ACTH, α-MSH, and β-MSH which were correlated with the three granule types observed.—The fact that the papers containing the largest numbers of cases (Hachmeister, 1973a; Olivier et al., 1972) contained either tumors with or without Crooke cells rises the suspicion that differences in fixation might be involved although a third paper (Foncin et al., 1972) presented both tumor types at the same time.—The presence of a large number of follicles lined by secretory and not by agranular follicular cells (see page 25) was described in one case (Bergland and Torack, 1969a). There was no basic difference in the ultrastructure of adenomas in Cushing's and Nelson's syndrome in the cases of Saeger (1973c) as well as in our own material which will be presented below.

Our own material was obtained from one case of Cushing's syndrome, two cases of Nelson's syndrome, and one case of Addison's disease with a pituitary adenoma. We will present the findings of the first three cases together because no Crooke cells have been observed in a total of five biopsies, whereas they were present in large numbers in the fourth case.

The patient with Cushing's disease underwent pituitary irradiation and subsequent subtotal removal of the hyperplastic adrenals at the age of 16 years. The skull X-rays showed a small sella throughout the whole course of the disease. A stereotaxic biopsy (no. 1/68) and electrocoagula-

Table 12. *Ultrastructural Findings in 27 Cases of Cushing's Syndrome Reported in the Literature*

Author(s)	Number of cases	Crooke cells	Granule size (mμ)
Bergland and Torack, 1969a	1	present	100–400
Foncin and Le Beau, 1963; Foncin, 1971	1	absent	120–180
Foncin *et al.*, 1972	2	one present one absent	180–500 120–180
Hachmeister, 1973a	10	absent	150–200
Olivier *et al.*, 1972	11	present	3 classes: –100, 200, 300–400
Porcile and Racadot, 1966	2	present	average 300

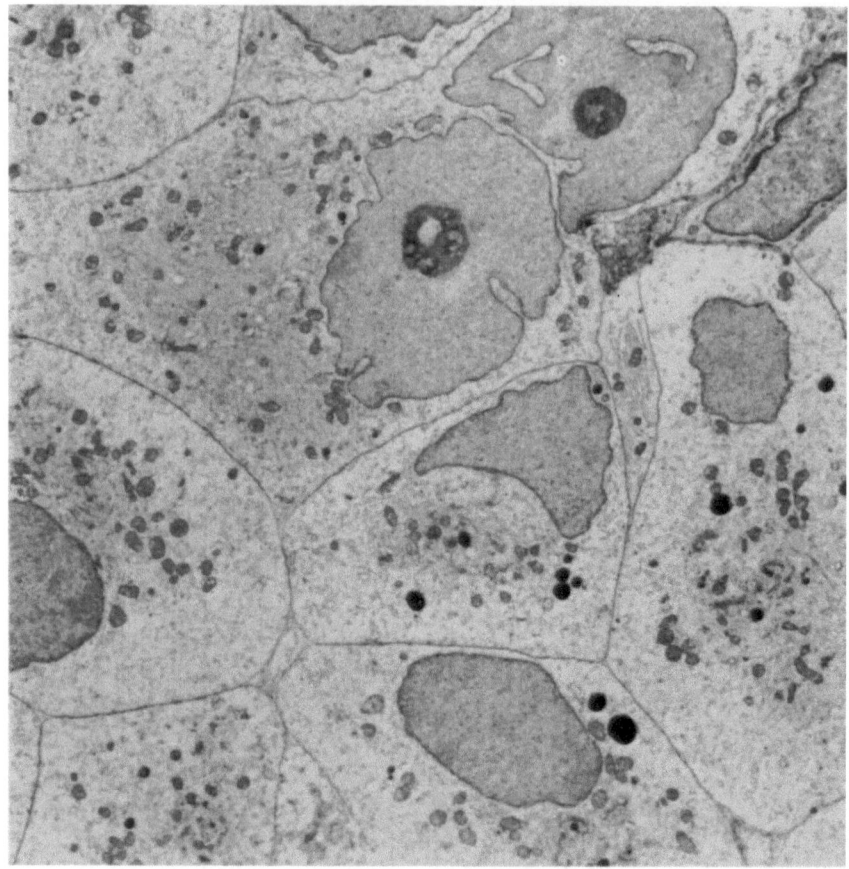

Fig. 37. Nelson syndrome: Polygonal cells with polymorphic nuclei demonstrating only few electron dense secretory granules. Presence of many large lipid bodies. A large part of the cytoplasm is occupied by an ill defined, fibrillary material. Case 10/74, osmium, ×3,900

tion of a pituitary micro-adenoma (Landolt and Siegfried, 1969) were performed because of continuing increased steroid production associated with slight hyperpigmentation. A second pituitary biopsy (no. 5/69) and sterotaxic yttrium[90] implantation were performed one year later.—The first patient with Nelson's syndrome underwent total adrenalectomy with subsequent cortisone substitution (37.5 mg cortisone acetate per day) in 1969 at the age of 41 years because of Cushing's disease. The adrenals were hyperplastic. She presented increased pigmentation and oculomotor palsy in 1970 and underwent a transfrontal, partial removal of a pituitary adenoma (biopsy no. 4/70) with postoperative X-ray

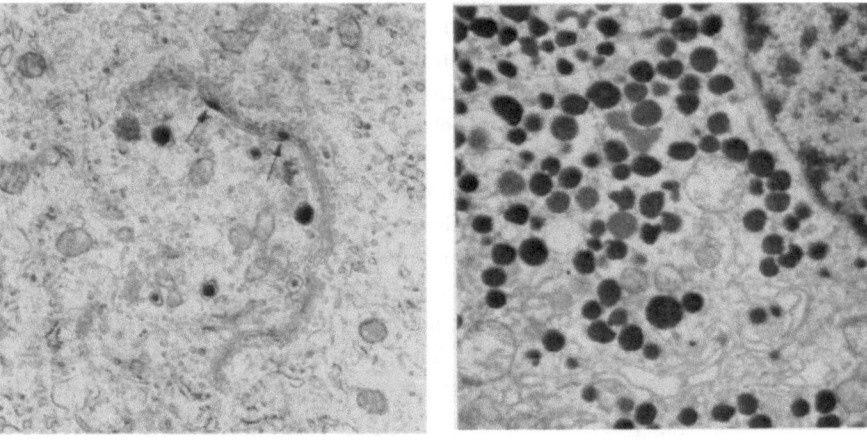

Fig. 38   Fig. 39

Fig. 38. Cushing syndrome: Golgi cisterns containing electron dense, spindle shaped accumulations of secretory material (arrows) surrounded by some few secretory granules and ill defined fibrillary material. Case 1/68, osmium, × 10,200

Fig. 39. Cushing syndrome: Adenoma cell loaded with numerous secretory granules showing varying electron density. Same patient as Fig. 38, biopsy obtained from second operation one year after first one and fixed with glutaraldehyde-osmium. Case 5/69, glutaraldehyde-osmium, × 9,100

therapy (4,000 rad local dose). She was operated upon a second time in 1971 because of tumor recurrence (biopsy no. 16/71).—Total extirpation of both hyperplastic adrenals was performed in the third patient because of Cushing's disease in 1962 at the age of 21 years. Since than she needed total cortisone substitution with 37.5 mg cortisone acetate per day. Increased pigmentation and bitemporal hemianopsia were observed in 1970. A transfrontal, subtotal removal of a pituitary adenoma (no. biopsy available) with postoperative X-ray therapy were performed. There was no change in intensity of pigmentation in spite of this. A transsphenoidal operation of an intrasellar tumor regrowth (suspected because of increased headaches) was performed in 1974 (biopsy no. 10/74).

In these three cases the ultrastructural examination of four tumor biopsies fixed directly in osmium shows almost identical findings (biopsies 1/68, 4/70, 16/71, 10/74). Strikingly different results are obtained from glutaraldehyde-osmium fixed and epon embedded (biopsy 5/69) or formalin-picric acid fixed and GMA embedded material (biopsy 10/74).— The tumors fixed with osmium alone consist essentially of a dense accumulation of oval, polygonal, or stellate cells with relatively scanty cytoplasm (Fig. 37). The nuclei are oval with some indentations in two

cases and polymorphic in another patient. All of them had been irradiated previously. The case with signs of invasive growth into the cavernous
sinus shows monomorphic nuclei in both biopsies. Nuclear polymorphism
also was of no value for determination of tumor growth character or
the influence of previous radiotherapy (see also pages 34 and 51).

The cytoplasm contains few organelles. The cells therefore look
empty. There are some mitochondria and few dispersed cisterns of the
RER. The Golgi complex usually is well developed. The cisterns are
regular and contain spindle shaped accumulations of electron dense material (Fig. 38), which is characteristic for this type of adenoma. It has
never been observed in cases with acromegaly, amenorrhea-galactorrhea,
or endocrine inactive adenomas. The electron dense material is strictly
confined to the interior of the cisterns and is therefore probably related
to the secretory product. Some secretory granules presenting an electron
dense core and a clearly separated membrane usually are present in the
Golgi region. They are otherwise extremely rare. Some irregular membranous profiles also can be recognized in the cytoplasm.

This picture of "empty" cells is completely changed by the use of
fixation media which contain aldehydes. Glutaraldehyde and osmium
fixed material shows an accumulation of secretory granules exhibiting
various degrees of electron density (Fig. 39) with irregular outlines and
diameters of 200–500 mμ. Formalin-picric acid fixation with subsequent
methacrylate embedding also demonstrates an abundance of granules
(Fig. 40) in the same tissue which lacks secretory products after direct
osmium fixation (Fig. 37). A similar behaviour has been described for the
predominant cell type of the pars intermedia of experimental animals
(see page 29), which usually has been associated with MSH production.
This differs from the assumption that MSH producing cells are the pre-
cursors of Crooke cells. Therefore it cannot yet be decided if the adenomas
of this group without Crooke cells produce MSH or ACTH. Another
interpretation might be that the pathological granules of ACTH producing adenomas are less resistent to osmium fixation than the normal
ACTH granules because of an abnormal molecular structure.

Pictures similar to those presented have been obtained from an
experimental rat pituitary tumor producing large quantities of ACTH
(Pelletier et al., 1971). The cells contained an undifferentiated RER, few
Golgi cisterns, few secretory granules with a diameter of 150–200 mμ,
and numerous lysosomes. The cells looked "empty" because of a small
content of organelles. No Crooke cells were observed.

The fourth case in our series is rather unique because it probably
represents the first case of long standing Addison's disease with a large
pituitary adenoma reported in the literature. Krause (1923) was the only
one to report a patient with Addison's disease demonstrating numerous,

adenoma-like, chromophobe cell hyperplasias of various dimensions in the pituitary.

Our patient (biopsy no. 43/73) suffered from bilateral coxitis and spondylitis of tuberculous origin at the age of two years and underwent several surgical procedures because of this between the age of two and six years. The diagnosis of Addison's disease of probable tuberculous origin was made at the age of 52 years. Adynamia and abnormal

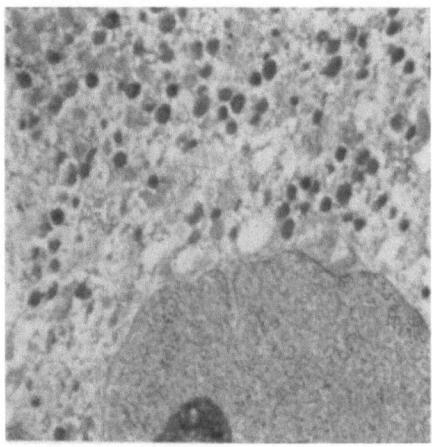

Fig. 40. Nelson syndrome: Numerous secretory granules with varying electron density can be visualized with formalin-picric acid fixation, embedding in methacrylate, and staining with osmium. Note difference to Fig. 37 obtained from same tumor but treated with direct osmium fixation. Case 10/74, formalin-picric acid, × 8,900

skin pigmentation disappeared after the institution of an appropriate substitution therapy (37.5 mg cortisone acetate per day and 50 mg desoxycorticosterone once per month as microcrystal injection). The patient noticed slowly increasing visual difficulties first in the right eye and later in the left eye as well as increased skin pigmentation at the age of 64 years. She ultimately became blind in the right eye and demonstrated temporal hemianopsia in the left eye. The neuroradiological examination showed a large supra-, intra-, and infrasellar pituitary adenoma. The endocrinological work-up demonstrated decreased gonadotropin and as well as normal TSH secretion. The plasma ACTH was increased to 2,000 pg/ml (normal basal values less than 50 pg/ml). This value could not be diminished by increased doses of cortisone. The large solid tumor was removed through a transsphenoidal approach. Vision increased and skin pigmentation decreased after surgery.

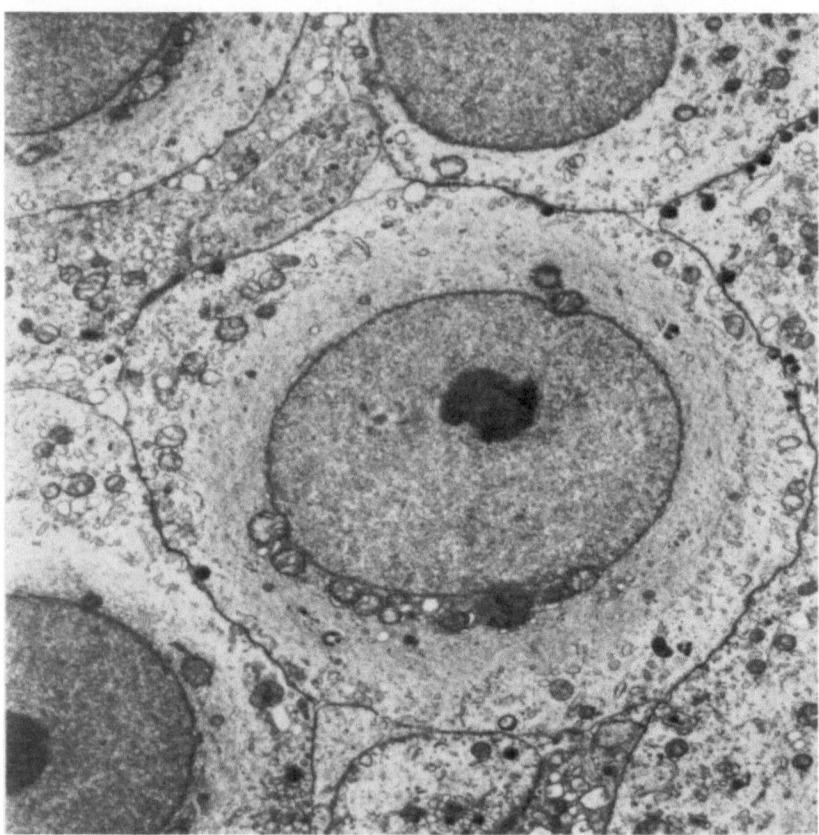

Fig. 41. Addison's disease: Accumulation of typical Crooke's cells in pituitary adenoma. The centrally placed nuclei are surrounded by a first
thin layer of cell organelles (mitochondria, vesicles, lysosomes) followed
by a layer of densely interwoven filaments in which some few organelles
are included, and a second layer of organelles. Secretory granules are usually
located beneath the cell membrane. Case 43/73, osmium, × 8,300

The ultrastructural examination of this corticotropic adenoma shows
that the tumor consists of large, round cells with centrally located round
or oval nuclei (Fig. 41). The nucleoli are prominent. The nuclei are
surrounded by a few organelles and a zone of densely interwoven filaments with a diameter of about 7 mμ (Fig. 42). This zone is identical
to a circular hyaline area seen in light micrographs. Another layer of
cell organelles containing most of the electron dense secretory granules is
located between the filaments and the cell membrane. The limitation of
space causes a dense accumulation of mitochondria, vesicles, small cisterns of the RER, free ribosomes, lysosomes, lipid bodies and centrioles.

The secretory granules are smaller in the zone near the nucleus whereas the larger ones are situated near the cell membrane. The granule diameter varies between 60 and 400 mμ with an average of 200 mμ (Fig. 43). These values are about 100 mμ below those found by Porcile and Racadot (1966). Some cells contain one extremely large or numerous smaller vacuoles (Fig. 44).

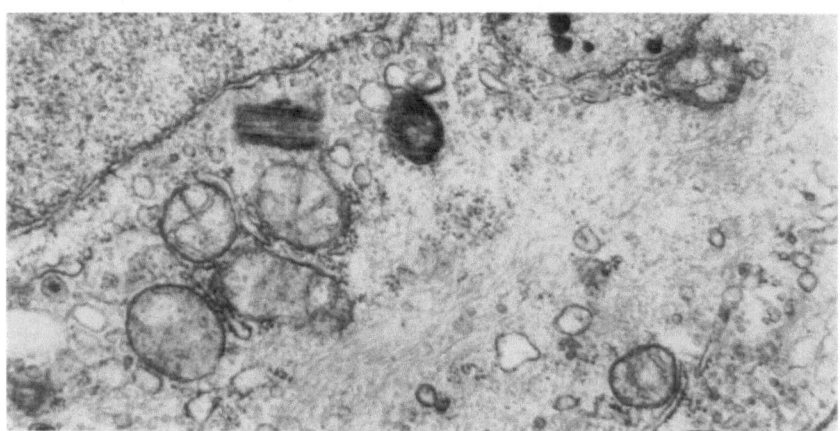

Fig. 42. Addison's disease: Detail showing nucleolus and nuclear membrane in upper left, mitochondria, vesicles, ribosomes, secretory granules, and centriole enclosed by irregularly arranged filaments in Crooke's cell. Case 43/73, osmium, × 30,000

The presence of typical Crooke cells in this adenoma suggests that the tumor is derived from the basophil cells of the former pars intermedia. The ACTH determination in this patient has been performed with anti-bodies for the sequence of the amino acids 1 to 24 of human ACTH which excludes the presence of α-MSH or β-MSH with a high degree of probabil-ity. The presence of ACTH in this particular tumor is not in accordance with the current concepts of hormone distribution in normal and neo-plastic pituitary tissue as discussed above.

We do not think that this is a reactive pituitary adenoma in a case of Addison's disease due to hormonal inbalance because the patient received an appropriate substitution therapy during the 12 years before the appearance of the pituitary neoplasm. Considering in additon the com-plete absence of similar cases in the literature we have to classify the observed syndrome as a coincidence of two extremely rare diseases: Addison's disease and a pituitary neoplasm which would have caused a Cushing's syndrome in a previously normal patient. Beta 1 basophils otherwise have been found to be significantly decreased in patients with

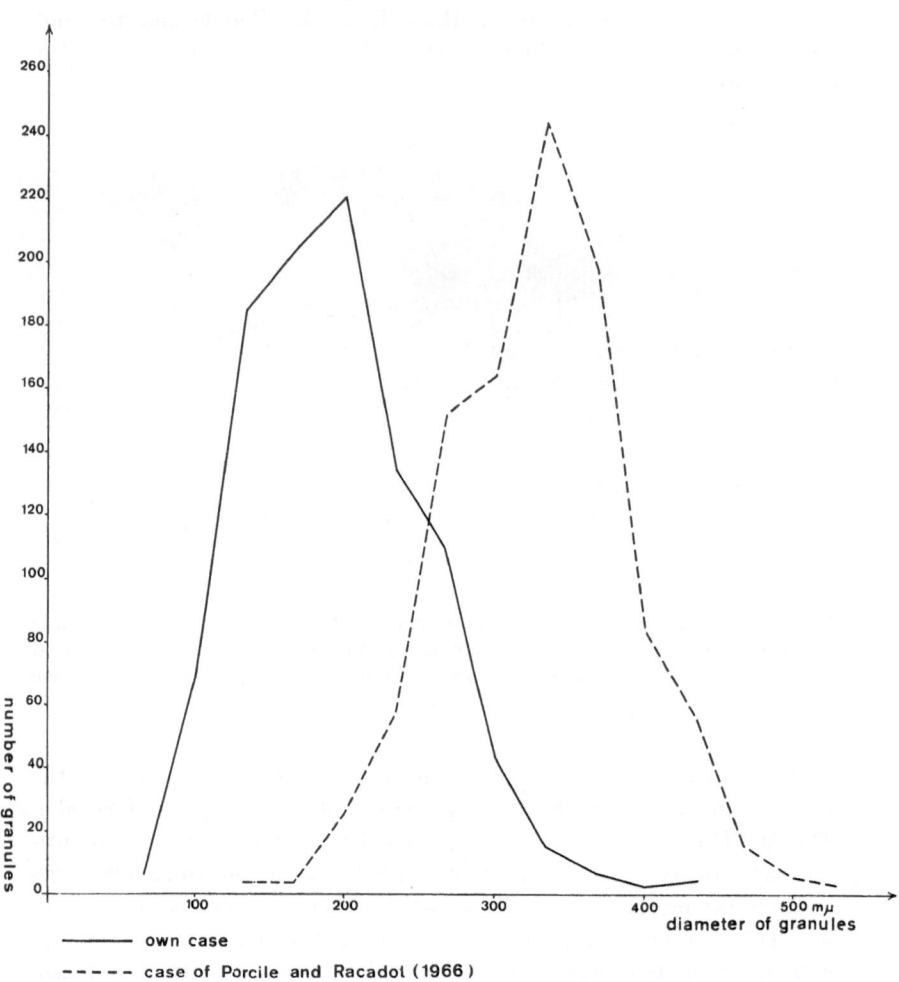

Fig. 43. Granule distribution curves of case with Crooke's cell adenoma in Addison's disease compared with case of Porcile and Racadot (1966) demonstrating Cushing's syndrome

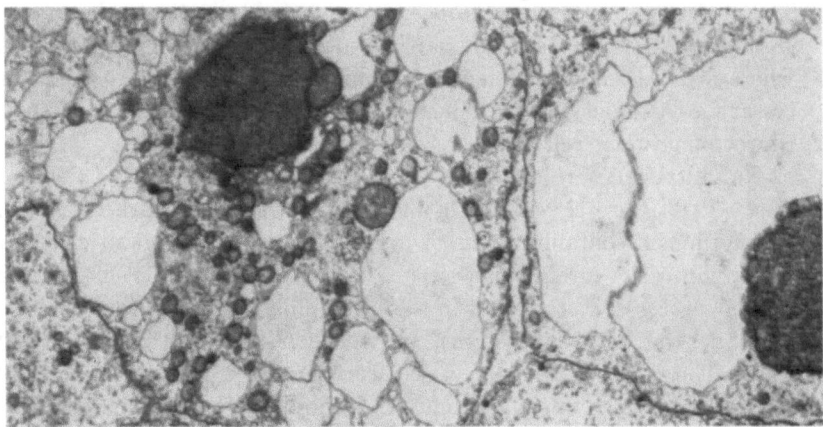

Fig. 44. Addison's disease: Cells with accumulation of numerous small or few large vesicles occupying large part of cytoplasm with some few intermingled organelles. Case 43/73, osmium, × 9,400

adrenal insufficiency (Ezrin and Murray, 1963). This tumor was not present prior to the destruction of the adrenals in the contrast to the pituitary adenomas in Nelson's syndrome.

4 d) Thyrotropic Adenomas of the Pituitary Gland

Thyrotropic adenomas of the pituitary gland are extremely rare. The literature contains only reports of single cases, and we do not have a similar case in our own series.—The following account of the literature includes only cases with thyroid disorders accompanied by a pituitary adenoma proven either by surgical biopsy or autopsy. Cases with pituitary adenomas treated by radiotherapy in which no histological report is available will not be mentioned.—It is evident from the literature that there are two types of thyrotropic pituitary tumors. The first one is associated with hyperthyroidism of rather short duration whereas the second one occurs together with congenital or long standing, severe hypothyroidism.

We were able to locate eight cases of pituitary adenoma associated with Grave's disease (Albeaux-Fernet et al., 1955; Erdheim, 1910; Jackson, 1965; Kappeler, 1959; Linquette et al., 1969; Mornex et al., 1972; Nyhan and Green, 1964; Werner and Stewart, 1958). Three patients underwent successful surgical removal of the pituitary adenoma with subsequent disappearance of hyperthyroidism. There were one basophilic micro-adenoma and three cyanophilic and three chromophobe adenomas reported.

This difference in staining characteristics probably is due to the type of stain used. Routine procedures showed only chromophobe adenomas whereas more sophisticated tetrachrome staining techniques were necessary to demonstrate specifically the cyanophilic or thioninophilic, thyrotropic tumor cell granules.

The ultrastructure of only a single case has been reported (Mornex et al., 1972, Curé et al., 1972). This tumor showed marked cellular polymorphism containing cells of normal size as well as giant elements and a number of intermediary forms. A complex pattern of interwoven cellular processes was present in the pericapillary spaces. Abnormalities of mitochondria, Golgi cisterns, and nucleoli were noted in the giant cells. The cells contained few secretory granules with a diameter of 90–150 mµ, rarely up to 300 mµ. The capillary endothelial cells were characterized by the presence of tubular inclusions with a diameter of 22 mµ which were localized in the perinuclear cisterns. These inclusions correspond to our virus-like structures observed in cases with acromegaly (see page 48).

The second type of thyrotropic adenoma is seen in patients with congenital or usually long standing, severe thyroid insufficiency. A total of 10 cases has been found in the literature (Caughey and Lester, 1961; Justin-Besançon et al., 1959; Kappeler, 1959; Langeron et al., 1954, 1959; Melnyck and Greer, 1965; Ponté et al., 1968; Racadot and Peillon, 1966; Schultze, 1914; Wegelin, 1925). Five adenomas were labeled as chromophobe. Three as basophilic or cyanophilic, one as mixed basophilic-eosinophilic, and one as eosinophilic tumors. No reports concerning the ultrastructure of such a tumor has yet been published.

Adenomas of the first type combined with Grave's disease usually have been interpreted as primary lesions. The adenomas of the second type associated with myxoedema have been considered to represent secondary lesions due to chronic hypothalamic stimulation due to loss of negative feed-back mechanisms.

5. Pituitary Adenomas without Signs of Endocrine Activity: The So-called "Chromophobe Adenomas"

The vast majority of pituitary adenomas do not show clinical signs of hormone production but rather manifest their presence by production of hypopituitarism and signs of compression of the visual pathways. Different patient series show a wide range in the frequency of the various symptoms. Vision is affected in 57–98%, menstrual disturbances occur in 17–85%, impotency and loss of libido are reported in 39–73%, the basal metabolism is decreased in 26–80%, and adrenal insufficiency is seen in 39–70% of the cases (Bakay, 1950; Davidoff and Feiring, 1948; Heimbach, 1959; Michard, 1958; Mundinger and Riechert, 1967). The variations in reported symptoms usually are interpreted as manifestations of the tumor size with variable compression of the optic system and destruction of the normal pituitary function.—These tumors usually are reported as "chromophobe adenomas" because routine histology fails to demonstrate stainable secretory granules. The term "chromophobe" therefore has been used as equivalent to "without signs of endocrine activity". This conclusion is not correct. We have demonstrated that HGH producing adenomas can contain only few granules in the case of rapid hormone discharge. Prolactin producing adenomas need special staining techniques for the demonstration of their granule content. We will show in the following chapter that the eosinophilic oncocytomas do not show any signs of hormone production. We suggest therefore that the term "chromophobe adenoma" should not be used in the description of clinical and pathological conditions. It should be replaced by "endocrine inactive adenoma". This term has the minor disadvantage of consisting of two words, but it fits the clinical entity much better. The following chapters will describe the ultrastructural types of endocrine inactive pituitary adenomas which can be differentiated.

5 a) Oncocytoma

Oncocytes are epithelial cells with a swollen appearance caused by an accumulation of minute granules of equal size which are stained by acid dyes. The nuclei are often dense and somewhat shrunken and therefore have been described as pycnotic. They demonstrate some degree of polymorphism. The word oncocyte was derived from the Greek term for "swollen" and introduced by Hamperl (1931, 1933) for these peculiar cells found in the normal salivary glands and some tumors of the parotid gland.—Finely granulated, swollen cells had been described before in the parathyroid (Erdheim, 1904), in the thyroid in Grave's disease (Askanazy, 1898) and in the large cell multifollicular adenoma (Langhans, 1907), and in the papillary cystadenoma lymphomatosum of the parotid (Warthin, 1929). Hamperl (1937, 1962a) critically reviewed the literature and his own material. He concluded that oncocytomas were the consequence of a persistent transformation (direct metaplasia, granular degeneration, modification) of epithelial cells of different organs indicating exhaustion occurring with age or after excessive functional stress. The Hürthle cells (Hürthle, 1894) do not belong to this group since the parafollicular cells of the thyroid show differences in light microscopy (Hamperl, 1950) and ultrastructure (Ekholm, 1964). This view has been opposed by Feldman et al. (1972) who think that Hürthle cells belong to the oncocyte group.

The oncocytic transformation of epithelial cells has been described in the normal salivary gland, the parathyroid, the thyroid, the kidney, the adrenal gland, the Fallopian tube, and the liver (for review see Hamperl, 1962a). This transformation also may occur in cells of both benign and malignant tumors of the organs enumerated. Since the capacity of the affected cells to multiply is preserved with oncocytic transformation, oncocytes themselves may form hyperplastic growths or even whole tumors. It is only for such tumors that the collective name oncocytoma is appropriate (Hamperl, 1962b).

The ultrastructure of oncocytes was first elucidated in the case of the oxyphil cells of the parathyroid (Elliott and Arhelger 1966; Lange, 1961; Rhodin, 1963; Roth, 1962; Roth et al., 1962; Trier, 1958). The cells contain innumerable, densely packed, partially abnormal mitochondria; several Golgi cisterns; an extremely reduced RER, and very few secretory granules. The accumulated mitochondria are responsible for the staining characteristics of the cells (Roth et al., 1962). The ultrastructure of oncocytes and oncocytomas since has been described in the parotid gland (Balogh and Roth, 1965; Hübner et al., 1965; Kay and Still, 1973; Tandler, 1966a, b; Tandler and Hoppel, 1972, Tandler and Shipkey, 1964; Tandler et al., 1970), lacrimal gland (Radnót and Lapis, 1970), thyroid (Feldman et al., 1972; Heimann et al., 1973), and lung (Fechner and Bentinck, 1973). These papers show that the ultrastructure of the oncocytes and oncocytomas in all organs mentioned remains basically unchanged and is characterized by the enormously increased number of structurally altered mitochondria.

In spite of the fact that the occurrence of oncocytes and oncocytomas has been suspected (Hamperl 1962a), the proof of their existence in the pituitary gland has been particularly difficult because of the presence of a mixture of various grades of chromophobe and eosinophil cells in the normal anterior lobe. Only electron microscopy has been able to establish the proof of their existence in the normal gland (Paiz and Hennigar, 1970). The same is true of pituitary oncocytomas. The descriptions of the

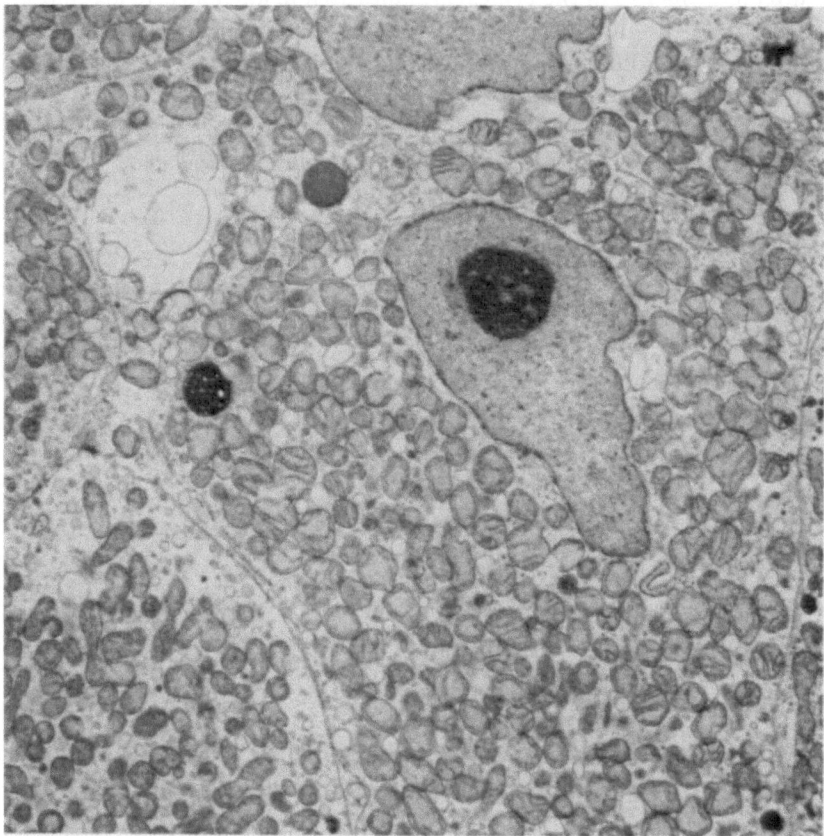

Fig. 45. Oncocytoma: Compact accumulation of adenoma cells with compact, somewhat irregular nucleus showing prominent nucleolus. The cytoplasm is filled with an abnormal number of mitochondria, some lipid droplets, and vesicles. Case 25/71, osmium, ×6,800

first two cases appeared almost simultaneously (Kovacs and Horvath, 1973; Landolt, 1973, 1974a; Landolt and Oswald, 1973).—We have now been able to collect a total of four cases in our own material. We are unaware of the publication of any additional observations prior to this report.

Light microscopy demonstrates that the tumors consist of solid epithelial cell strands which are in close apposition to capillaries forming a slightly irregular, trabecular network. The cells are usually oval and have a swollen appearance. The somewhat polymorphic nuclei show a densely structured chromatin producing the picture of pyknosis. The cytoplasm is occupied by innumerable, fine acidophilic granules which are much finer than the typical granules seen in adenomas of acromegalic patients. The difference is seen most clearly in phase contrast micrographs of osmium fixed and plastic embedded material (see Figs. 1, 2 of Landolt and Oswald, 1973).

Examination by electron microscopy demonstrates a dense accumulation of epithelial cells with only few capillaries and collagen fibrils.

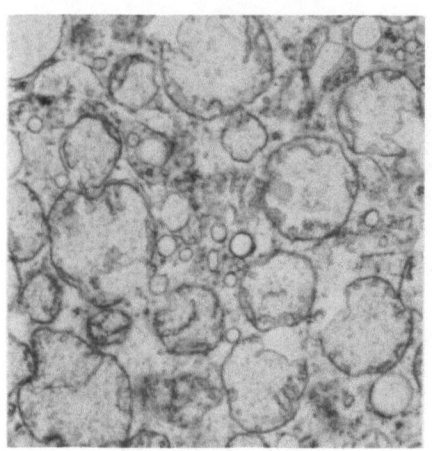   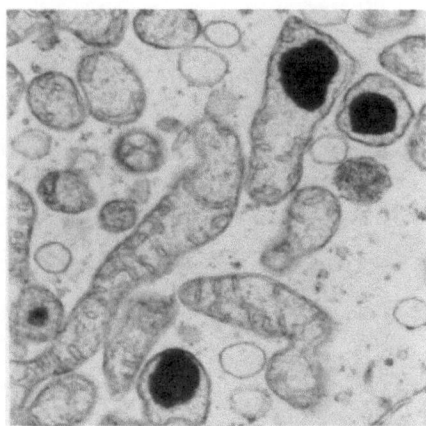

Fig. 46   Fig. 47

Fig. 46. Oncocytoma: Abnormal mitochondria showing deformed and rudimentary cristae and finely granular matrix.   Case 25/71, osmium, × 16,300

Fig. 47. Oncocytoma: Mitochondria with varying degree of structural alterations and electron dense inclusion bodies.   Case 25/71, osmium, × 16,200

The cells are usually polygonal or oval, rarely stellate, with diameters of up to 15 μ. The cell boundaries are not obvious because of a dense accumulation of cell organelles. A large part of the cell body is occupied by the evenly structured, often polymorphic and intended nucleus containing a prominent nucleolus (Fig. 45). The cytoplasm of the cells is densely packed with innumerable round or oval, sometimes distorted mitochondria (Fig. 46). The mitochondrial structure in most instances is abnormal. The pattern of cristae is disturbed. They form circles, elongated sacs, clubs, arcades, and three-dimensional tubular networks. The matrix is finely granular and occupies the major part of the volume. The intermembrane spaces may be distended locally. Occasional dense inclusions can be found (Fig. 47). Few free ribosomes and some smooth surfaced vesicles can be seen (Fig. 46). Lipid inclusions are numerous

(Fig. 45). Golgi cisterns and lysosomes are frequent (Fig. 48). Centrioles can be observed in their vicinity. Secretory granules with dense cores are rare in the typical oncocytoma cell. They measure 100–240 mμ in diameter. The RER is characteristically absent. The structure of the capillaries as well as their relation to the adenoma cells is unremarkable except for the paucity of the vascular supply.

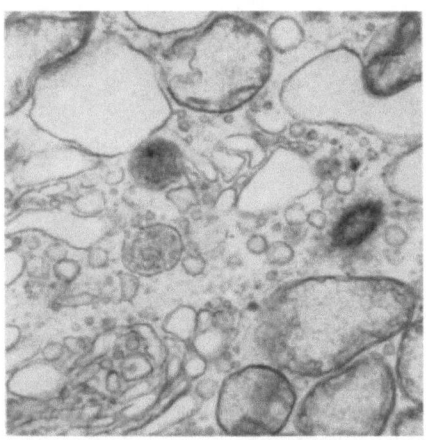

Fig. 48. Oncocytoma: Lysosomes, Golgi cisterns, vesicles, and centriole accumulated between deformed mitochondria. Case 25/71, osmium, × 21,800

Two of the four specimens examined consisted almost entirely of typical oncocytes whereas the remaining two examples showed many intermediate forms with fewer mitochondria and more frequent dense granules (Fig. 49) similar to the case presented by Kovacs and Horvath (1973). This leads to the question concerning the stage at which the oncocytic transformation of the tumor takes place. 1. It is possible that the metaplasia occurs in certain cells in a pre-existing adenoma which inherited the capability to form oncocytes from the normal tissue. This leads to a tumor containing cells in various stages of transformation. 2. The metaplasia can occur at the very beginning of the tumor growth. The oncocytes retain the capability of cell division (Tandler *et al.*, 1970) giving origin to a tumor composed exclusively of this cell species (Hamperl, 1962 b).

The ultrastructural characteristics clearly differentiate the pituitary oncocytomas from the other pituitary adenomas without signs of endocrinological activity *i.e.*, the endocrine inactive adenomas (see Chapter 5 b). The question concerning a clinical or biological difference of this tumor type is not yet answered.—Our own four cases suggest that there are no fundamental but rather gradual differences present. The onco-cytomas seem to occur mostly in the older age group. The age of our own patients at the time of surgery was 46, 47, 53, and 56 years, respectively, giving an average of 50.5 years. The average age of 48 cases of the usual endocrine inactive adenomas was 44.7 years. There are three males and one female. Their main complaint concerned visual difficulties. All pa-

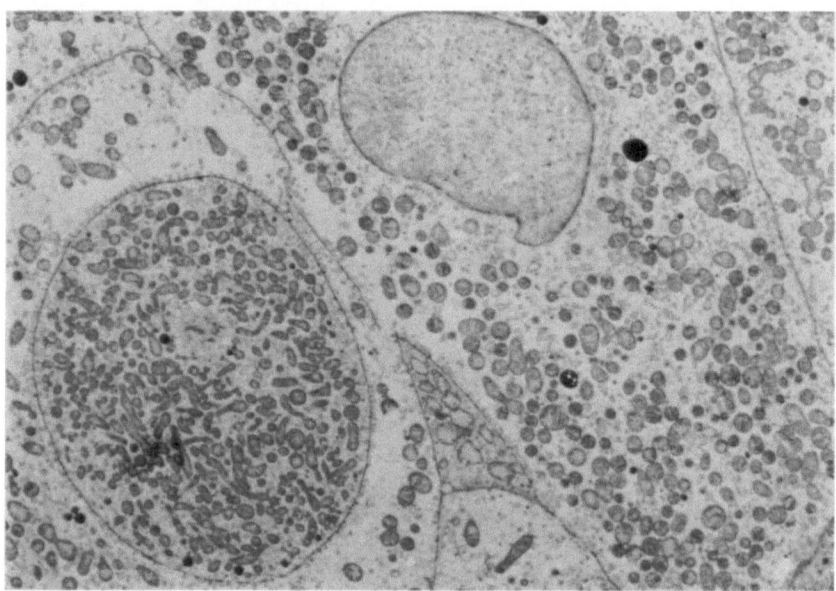

Fig. 49. Oncocytoma: Adenoma with cells demonstrating less uniform degree of mitochondria alteration. Some cells contain an enormously increased number of mitochondria whereas the number is in the normal range in others. Case 38/73, osmium, × 3,900

tients showed severe visual impairment (visual losses of 46, 74, 91, and 97% according to the Committee on Medical Rating, 1958) grouping all except one in the stage III of Svien and Colby (1967). The endocrinolo-gical symptoms were of minor importance. Two male patients admitted loss of sexual potency only after direct questioning whereas one patient claimed to function normally. The female patient was in the postmeno-pausal stage at the time of tumor occurrence. The thyroid function was normal in three and decreased in one patient. The adrenal function was normal in two and borderline decreased in the remaining two patients.

The duration of symptoms was short in two patients (two and three months). Both showed oncocytomas with numerous intermediary cells. The two adenomas consisting entirely of oncocytes presented a much longer duration of symptoms reaching 6 years in one and 13 years in the other patient. It has to be mentioned that the second patient suffered from a recurrent tumor which had caused symptoms two years before the first operation. The review of the light microscopy slides of both biopsies showed identical features. The examination of additional cases is required to determine whether this difference in duration of the pre-operative symptoms reflects a true ultrastructural characteristic based on differing biological properties.—It is interesting to note that the two patients with rapidly progressive symptoms complained of headaches whereas the other two did not. Signs of invasion into the cavernous sinus have not been seen in the case of Kovacs and Horvath (1973) nor in our own four patients.

The growth of at least some oncocytomas is very slow when compared to other pituitary adenomas. Symptoms of recurrence appeared in 95% of Cushing's series within five years. None was observed after eight years (German and Flanigan, 1964). The signs of regrowth appeared in our particular case only after a 13-year interval.

Summarizing the above mentioned observations we can describe the following clinical features of pituitary oncocytomas: they occur mainly in patients older than 35 years who complain chiefly about visual disturb-ances. Careful inquiry and endocrinological work-up reveal only minor deficiencies. At least some of the tumors show an extremely slow growth rate.

Nothing is yet known about the X-ray sensitivity of pituitary onco-cytomas because of their recent description. Oncocytomas of the thyroid, parathyroid and parotid are judged to be insensitive or only moderately sensitive to X-ray therapy (Eneroth and Jacobsson, 1972; Russel et al., 1963; Tillinger, 1947). One of our cases showed a tumor recurrence in spite of conventional postoperative irradiation with a local tumor dose of 4,000 rads. Two of the remaining cases also received postoperative radiation therapy but one did not. A critical follow-up of the cases and the destiny of future patients will show if oncocytomas are an exception to the well known radiosensitivity of the ordinary endocrine pituitary adenoma (Ennuyer and Cheguillaume, 1958; German and Flanigan, 1964; Henderson, 1939; Mundinger and Riechert, 1967; Svien and Colby, 1967).

Since oncocytes occur in the normal tissue of older patients in other glands, it has been assumed that they represent transformations due to exhaustion and are biologically deficient (Fechner and Bentinck, 1973; Hamperl, 1937, 1962a; Tandler, 1966a). The mitochondrial hyperplasia therefore might be due to compensatory mechanisms. Biochemical studies on oncocytes have demonstrated that certain mitochondrial enzymes show increased function (Balogh and Cohen, 1961; Balogh and Roth, 1965; Tremblay and Pearse, 1959, 1960) and signs of loosely coupled states of oxidative phosphorylation reflecting an inefficient function (Shiefer *et al.*, 1968). This condition has been compared to a myopathy also showing increased numbers of mitochondria and signs of a deficient mitochondrial respiratory control (Luft *et al.*, 1962).

Signs of increased endocrine activity were present neither in the case of Kovacs and Horvath (1973) nor in our own four patients. Morphologically the cytoplasm of the tumor cells contained only rare secretory granules and did not display any ultrastructural features indicating enhanced protein synthesis. This finding is in accordance with the conclusion of previous investigators showing that no biosynthesis of thyroxine or thyroglobulin seems to occur in oxyphilic adenomas of the human thyroid (Heimann *et al.*, 1973). Hyperparathyroidism has been described in oxyphilic adenomas of the parathyroid (Purnell *et al.*, 1971; Roth, 1962).—No definite conclusion can be drawn from these descriptions since the adenomas of the parathyroid usually contain a mixture of chief cells, clear cells and oncocytes.

5 b) Endocrine Inactive Adenomas with Secretory Granules

Endocrine inactive adenomas with secretory granules form the largest group of pituitary neoplasms in our series. They are slightly less frequent in the literature than cases with acromegaly. We have been able to collect about 150 cases from a total of 19 papers published (Brucher *et al.*, 1970; Foncin, 1971; Hachmeister, 1973a, b; Hirano *et al.*, 1972; Kuromatsu, 1967; Lewis and Van Noorden, 1974; Luse, 1961; Mackay *et al.*, 1973; Nyström, 1973; Oliva *et al.*, 1966; Pelletier, 1971; Peillon *et al.*, 1971; Schechter, 1973a; Schelin, 1962; Tomiyasu *et al.*, 1973; Wechsler and Hossmann, 1965; Zambarano *et*, *al.* 1968). Almost every author has noted that this type of adenoma contains secretory granules and displays granule extrusion in spite of the complete absence of clinical signs of secretory activity. The reported granule size was generally smaller than that observed in acromegaly and corresponded more to the size seen in normal corticotrophs and gonadotrophs. Most authors concluded that abnormal substances were produced because of the lack of signs of hypergonadotropism or hypercorticism. The regular presence of secretory granules corresponded well to the results in the paper of McCormick and Halmi (1971); they demonstrated an absence of chromophobe adenomas in a series of 145 pituitary neoplasms. There were 59% acidophilic, 18.4% basophilic, and 15.8% mixed adenomas. The remaining 6.8% showed signs of autolysis and could not be classified. Only 3% of the acidophilic and 7% of the basophilic adenomas showed signs of acromegaly and Cushing's disease, respectively. The nature of the secretion product remained unrecognized in the large majority of the

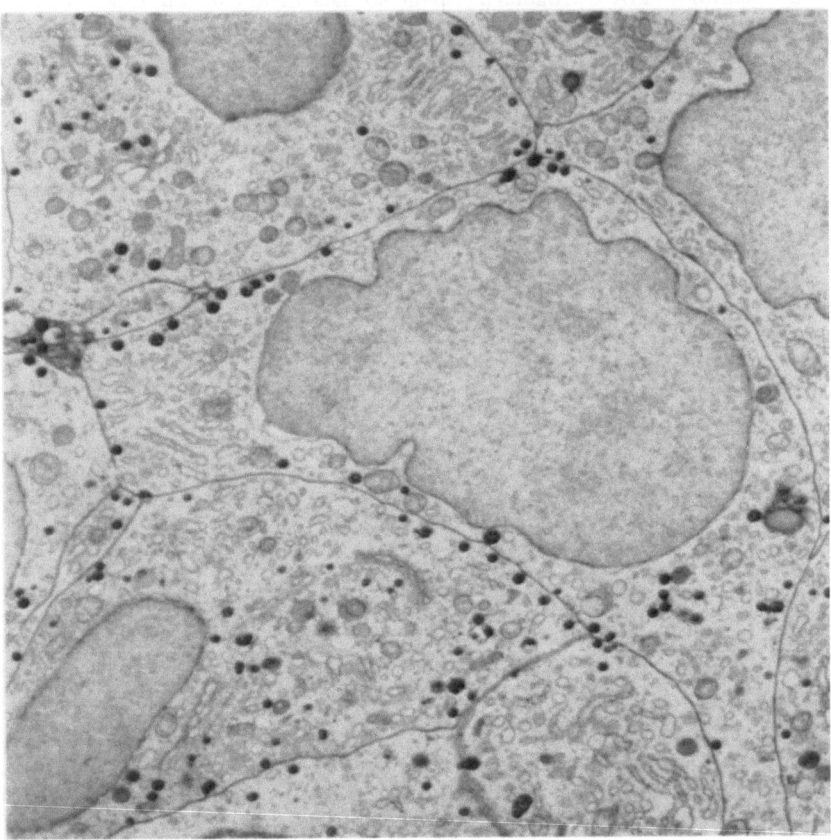

Fig. 50. Peillon-Racadot syndrome: Polygonal adenoma cells with somewhat polymorphic nuclei. Numerous Golgi cisterns and sacs of the RER as
well as deformed secretory granules, lipid bodies, mitochondria, and some
lysosomes are located in the cytoplasm. Case 11/70, osmium, × 8,300

cases. These results of light microscopy as well as the fact that a variety
of granule types were found on ultrastructural examination suggested
that possibly a variety of substances might be produced.

Peillon and collaborators (1966) were the first to observe a chronologi-
cal relation between the estrogens treatment of amenorrheic female
patients and signs of pituitary tumor progression (increased headaches
or decreasing vision) in five out of eight cases with so called "chromophobe" adenomas. The histological examination showed signs of tumor
proliferation as well as hemorrhages and mitoses. Five adenomas contained erythrosinophilic granules. The authors concluded that these adenomas probably secreted prolactin since prolactin secreting cells and tumors

are stimulated by estrogens (see page 20; Delthil and Julou, 1960; Racadot and Peillon, 1968).—The syndrome presented by a female patient with a pituitary neoplasm which is stimulated by estrogens administered for reinstitution of a menstrual cycle and which is associated with secondary amenorrhea in the absence of galactorrhea or other signs of endocrine activity will be called "Peillon-Racadot" syndrome. The Peillon-Racadot syndrome is a Forbes-Albright syndrome without galactorrhea.

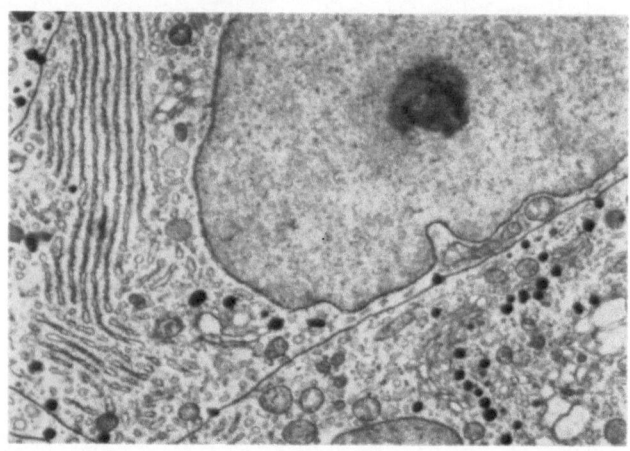

Fig. 51. Peillon-Racadot syndrome: Detail of adenoma cell demonstrating elaborate secretory organelles as highly developped RER and numerous Golgi cisterns. Presence of deformed secretory granules. Case 11/70, osmium, × 8,100

The effect of estrogen administration can be used as clinical test for prolactin secreting tumors. But we will demonstrate below that there is a considerable number of false negative results. The negative cases can be detected only by the radioimmuno assay of prolactin performed in a blood sample.

Our series contains one case with a typical Peillon-Racadot syndrome. The patient suffered since the age of 28 years from secondary amenorrhea. She received in the subsequent eleven years a total of three courses of estrogen-progesterone medication. Each trial had to be stopped because of severe headaches, nausea, and vertigo which disappeared after discontinuing the treatment. She also suffered severe headaches from diplopia and a temporal visual field defect on the left eye during the last trial of medication at the age of 40 years. The headaches and diplopia disappeared after cessation of the therapy. The visual field defect increased later on and led ultimately to the discovery of the pituitary adenoma which was operated upon (biopsy no. 11/70). A fine erythro-

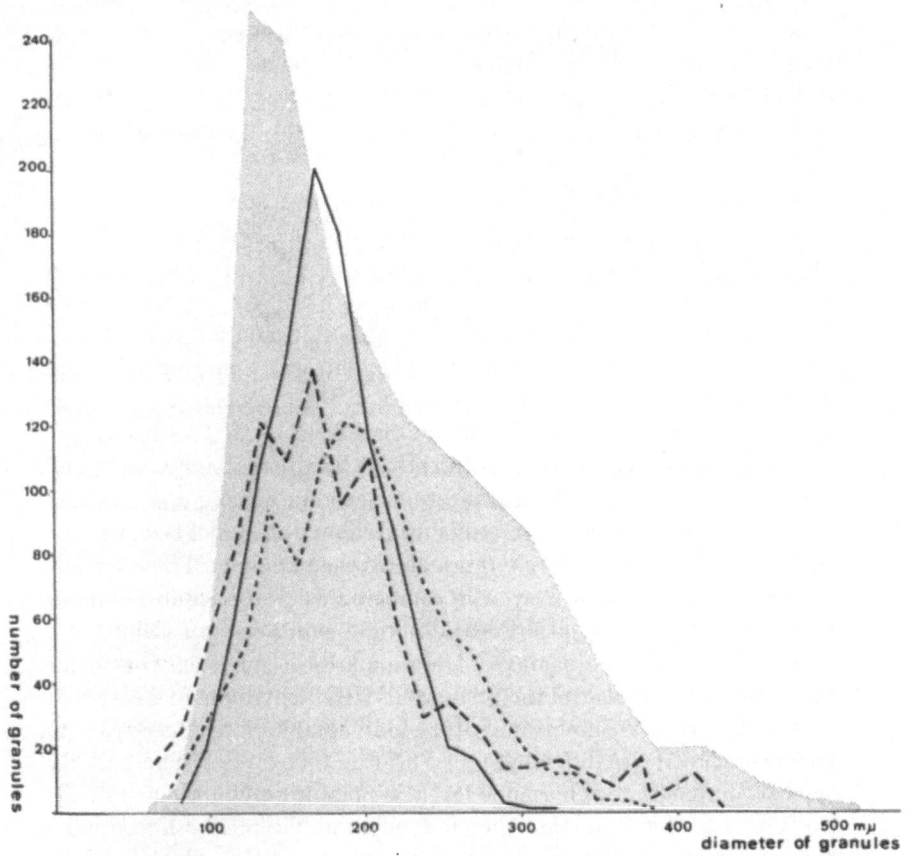

Fig. 52. Granule size distribution curves of one case with Peillon-Racadot syndrome (solid line) and two cases of seemingly endocrine inactive adenomas showing silent, enormously increased prolactin production (broken lines) compared with our cases with typical Forbes-Albright syndrome (shaded area)

sinophilic granulation was demonstrated with light microscopy. Routine staining methods had only shown a "chromophobe" adenoma.

The ultrastructural examination of the tumor shows that it consists of a dense accumulation of polygonal cells (Fig. 50) with polymorphic nuclei containing a homogenous chromatin structure. The cytoplasm is filled with an accumulation of numerous Golgi cisterns, an organized RER (Fig. 51), various lysosomes, vesicles, and mitochondria. A fair number of electron dense secretory granules can be seen dispersed in the cytoplasm. The granules have an average diameter of 175 mμ (Fig. 52, uninterrupted line). The larger granules often have irregular outlines.

This has been noted to be characteristic for the prolactin producing tumors of cases with Forbes-Albright syndrome (see page 53). These findings demonstrate an ultrastructural picture which is typical for cells engaged in active protein synthesis. This product is at least in part prolactin as demonstrated by the results of the histological examination and the typical case history.

Prolactin synthesis has been observed in two additional cases who neither presented the characteristic history of the Peillon-Racadot syndrome nor showed a galactorrhoea as in the Forbes-Albright syndrome. The two female patients, both of whom were 25 years of age, suffered from secondary amenorrhea since the age of 18 and 22 years, respectively. The presence of a pituitary adenoma was found in both cases during the evaluation performed because of the amenorrhea. No visual symptoms were noted. Both patients had been treated with estrogen-progesterone medications without ill effect. The function of the adrenals and thyroid as well as the gonadotropin excretion was normal in both cases. The serum prolactin determination showed values of 800 and more than 1,000 ng/ml, respectively (normal less than 25 ng/ml). These values are enormously increased even if compared with the results obtained from patients with a typical Forbes-Albright syndrome (see Table 10).

Initiation and maintenance of lactation are based not only on prolactin production but also on the presence of HGH, thyroxin, and corticoids as well. The relative importance of the individual hormones necessary for lactogenesis varies in different species (Cowie, 1966). We assume that this typical combination of hormone levels is present only in a few patients. The presence of galactorrhea therefore might only represent a rare symptom of pituitary neoplasms secreting prolactin. Accordingly, a large number of patients with adenomas of this type might escape our clinical observation. Another possible explanation for the absence of galactorrhea in the three cases presented in this chapter may be the secretion of abnormal prolactin molecules which still contain the antigenic amino acid sequence necessary for the radioimmuno assay but which no longer show any biological activity. This problem needs further investigation.

Routine histology shows a "chromophobe" adenoma in both patients presented above whereas erythrosine staining demonstrates the presence of scarce, pink granules in the adenoma cells.—The ultrastructural examination proves that the adenomas are engaged in active protein synthesis. The cells contain numerous Golgi complexes (Fig. 53), a large number of vesicles, and a well developed RER. The formation of annulate lamellae can be observed in one case (Fig. 54). Annulate lamellae are known to occur in oocytes and in embryonic and adult neoplastic tissues. The ultrastructure of a single lamella resembles the nuclear membrane. They are formed possibly from blebs of the outer membrane

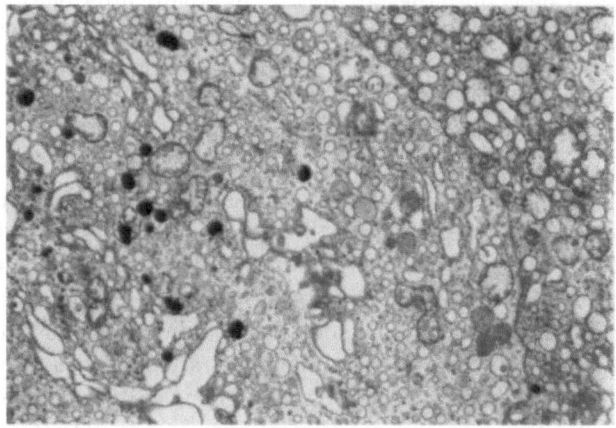

Fig. 53. Pituitary adenoma with clinically silent prolactin production: Presence of Golgi cisterns, well developed RER, and numerous deformed, electron dense, secretory granules. Case 70/73, osmium, ×6,000

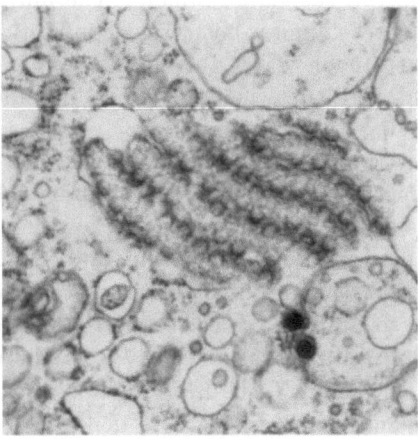

Fig. 54. Pituitary adenoma with clinically silent prolactin production: Formation of annulate lamellae in connection with RER (upper left corner). Case 70/73, osmium, ×21,800

of the nuclear envelope. In addition, they may result from reorganization or development of the RER. They probably are related to protein or peptide synthesis since they are present in rapidly growing tissues or cells engaged in protein secretion (for review see Wischnitzer, 1970). Their presence has been reported in a rapidly growing parathyroid adenoma (Elliott and Arhelger, 1966) but not previously in a pituitary tumor.

Secretory granules are less frequent than in the case with the Peillon-Racadot syndrome described above. Their size is the same as can be seen in the distribution curves in Fig. 52. All three curves coincide with the shadowed area representing the cases with Forbes-Albright syndromes. Furthermore the granules show the irregular outlines typical for the larger prolactin containing granules. We suggest therefore that the presence of the typical morphological pattern of a well developed RER and Golgi system, deformed granules, and absence of intracytoplasmic filaments characterizes a pituitary adenoma with possible prolactin production. These criteria are typical but are not obligatory since we have presented a tumor with proven prolactin secretion not showing this picture (Fig. 34).—The secretory activity index in the two adenomas is five in both cases. This number fits perfectly with the excessive serum prolactin levels found before surgery.

Gross degenerative changes in chromophobe adenomas are said to be unusual except in the very large tumors. The nutrition of the tumors usually is well preserved unless hemorrhagic infarction occurs secondary to rapid growth; strangulation of the blood supply with ischemia, necrosis, and hemorrhage occurs when the expanding adenoma has become impacted at the diaphragmatic notch (for review see Rovit and Fein, 1972). The ultrastructural examination of the sella contents in a case with massive hemorrhagic infaction of a pituitary adenoma (which had not caused any clinical symptoms before the apoplexy leading to sudden headaches, blindness on one eye and temporal hemianopsia on the other 18 days before surgery) shows only necrotic cells (Fig. 55). The individual cell remnants are separated from each other. The cytoplasmic constituents are swollen or destroyed leaving only some intact secretory granules. The nuclear chromatin structure is disrupted leaving only irregular spaces between some strands of electron dense material. Hemorrhagic infarction can also lead to cystic transformation of various parts of the adenomas (Kernohan and Sayre, 1956; Russell and Rubinstein, 1971); this can be seen in 17–30% of the cases with pituitary adenomas reported (Dott et al., 1925; Henderson, 1939; McLean, 1936; Paterson, 1948).

When calcification occurs in pituitary adenomas, it may be found either in the central portion or in the wall of a cyst. In a study of 285 of Cushing's verified adenomas Deery (1929) found 7% of the cases showing calcium shadows within or just above the sella turcica in the skull

X-ray. No constant factors (such as the type of adenoma, the duration of the disease, or the age of the patient) were found that might have influenced the development of calcifications. The same incidence of 7% was reported by McLean (1936). There was an incidence of only 3.2% in 345 cases examined by Lindgren and Di Chiro (1951). They concerned only "chromophobe" adenomas. Deery (1929) states that he had not seen

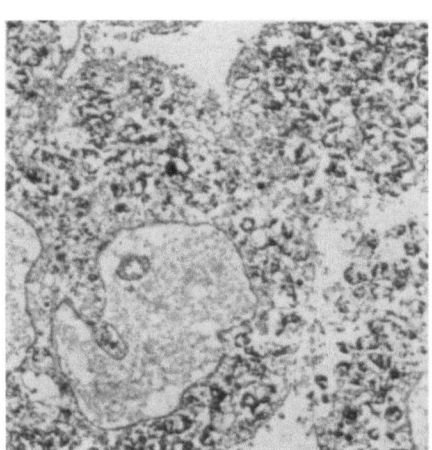 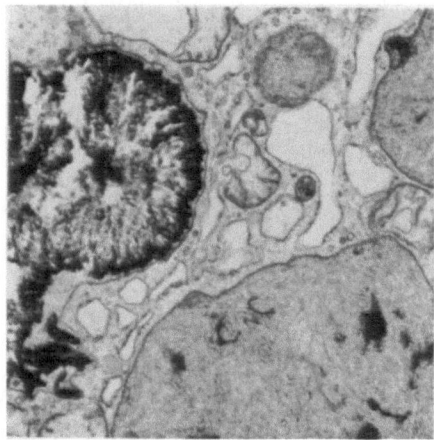

Fig. 55   Fig. 56

Fig. 55. Pituitary apoplexy: Biopsy of necrotic adenoma obtained 18 days after acute infarction showing separated, necrotic cell remnants. Case 26/71, osmium, × 9,400

Fig. 56. Pituitary adenoma with clinically silent prolactin production: Extracellular, spherical calcification (upper left) consisting of crystalline needles and intracellular fibrillar inclusion. Dilatation of cisterns of the RER. Case 32/73, osmium, × 14,800

calcifications in the histologic sections of the cases with positive X-ray findings. The presence of large calcispherites, which were similar to psammoma bodies, has been described in a few cases presenting usually a long history of the disease (Hastrup, 1966; Kraus, 1926, 1945; Russell and Rubinstein, 1971).

One of the two cases with prolactin producing adenoma without clinical signs of endocrine activity (no. 32/73) shows widespread foci of calcification. No calcifications had been present on the skull X-rays before surgery. Small, spherical accumulations of hydroxyapatite crystals can be seen in the extracellular space (Fig. 56). In addition the adenoma cells of this case contain dense bodies with fibrillar inclusions; such have not been found in any of the other cases examined. Similar

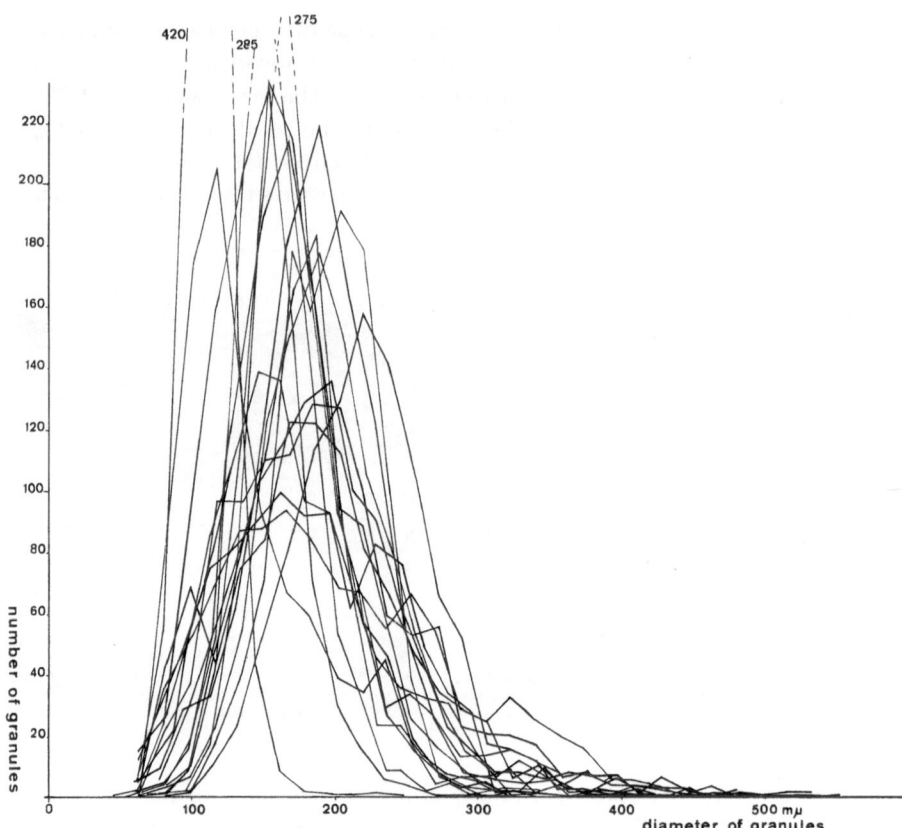

Fig. 57. Granule size distribution curves of 18 unselected cases with endocrine inactive pituitary adenomas. For further explanation see text

formations have been described by Tomiyasu and collaborators (1973) who interpreted them as being lysosomal in nature.

The remaining 45 cases demonstrate a variety of ultrastructural pictures which can be subdivided. This procedure is entirely hypothetical since no results of corresponding hormone determinations in the blood, tumor tissue, or culture media are available. Further observations and investigations will be necessary to elucidate the nature of the secretory products observed in these adenomas. The examination of the granule size distribution curves of 18 unselected cases from this group shows a picture which is much more uniform than, *e.g.*, in acromegaly (Fig. 57). The average diameter varies between 110 and 223 mμ compared with 130–350 mμ in acromegaly or 157–277 mμ in Forbes-Albright syndrome. The results demonstrate again that the granule size cannot be used as the only criterion for cell type identification in neoplasms as is done in

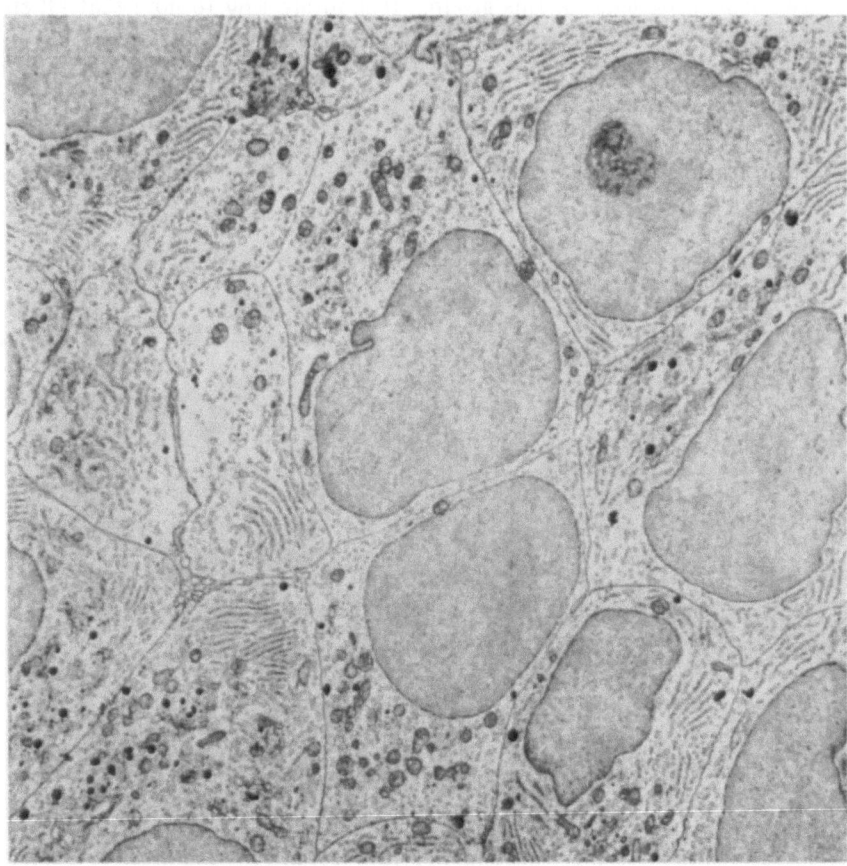

Fig. 58. Endocrine inactive pituitary adenoma: Polygonal cells with relatively large nuclei, an elaborate RER, well developed Golgi cisterns, and secretory granules giving the impression of an adenoma with active hormone production. Case 45/72, osmium, × 4,500

normal tissue. This fact also has been stressed by others (Mackay *et al.*, 1973; Schechter, 1973a; Schelin, 1962). Therefore other structural criteria have to be used for a possible classification.

We have noted above that in the major number of biopsies examined adenomas producing prolactin show secretory granules which are not round or slightly oval as in acromegaly but often deformed. Applying this criterion to the 45 cases in question, we find 6 cases with identical granules. Furthermore, these cases show a well developed RER and numerous Golgi cisterns (Figs. 58 and 59). Therefore they cannot be differentiated from prolactin producing adenomas. There were four male and two female patients in this group. It is interesting to note that all six patients complained about impotency, loss of libido, or amenorrhea as leading symptoms in spite of the fact that three adenomas were small and had not yet caused visual symptoms.

Another group of five patients (3 males, 2 females) show ultrastructural features corresponding exactly to the picture found in many acro-

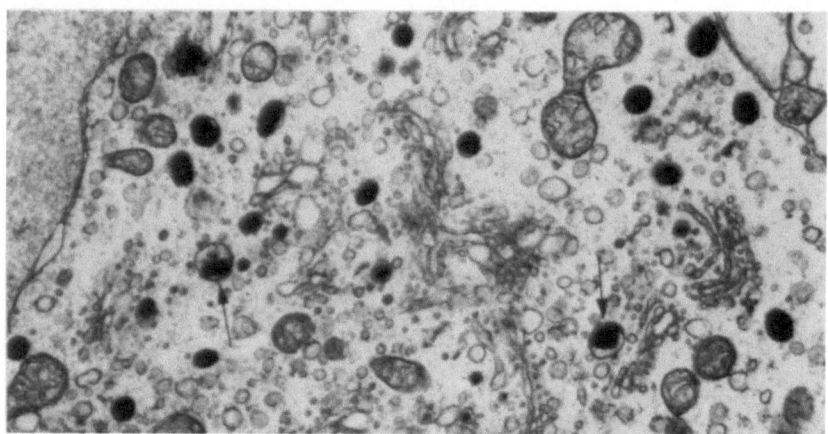

Fig. 59. Endocrine inactive pituitary adenoma: Accumulation of Golgi cisterns and deformed secretory granules similar to prolactin producing adenoma. Some lysosomes are engaged in hormone digestion (arrow). Case 22/71, osmium, ×17,600

megalic cases. The most prominent structures are circular areas of loosely interwoven filaments enclosing secretory granules, mitochondria, and empty vesicles (Fig. 60). The assumption that these tumors might produce HGH cannot be proven, for the patients showed the clinical symptoms of an endocrine inactive adenoma without signs of acromegaly. No HGH determinations were obtained.—Our assumption of HGH production by seemingly inactive tumors fits perfectly with the results of immunohistochemical examination of pituitary adenomas with enzyme-labelled antibodies by Kirsch and Nakane (1973). Several cases of their series identified clinically as "chromophobe" adenomas contained sparse granulations with positive reactions to anti-HGH.

The adenomas of two patients without signs of endocrine activity demonstrate the presence of numerous follicular cells with formation of abnormal and abortive follicles (Fig. 61). The cells are connected to each other by irregularly arranged desmosomes (Fig. 62). Numerous lysosomes can be detected in their cytoplasm. The cells do not contain secretory granules, but granulated cells not engaged in follicle formation are

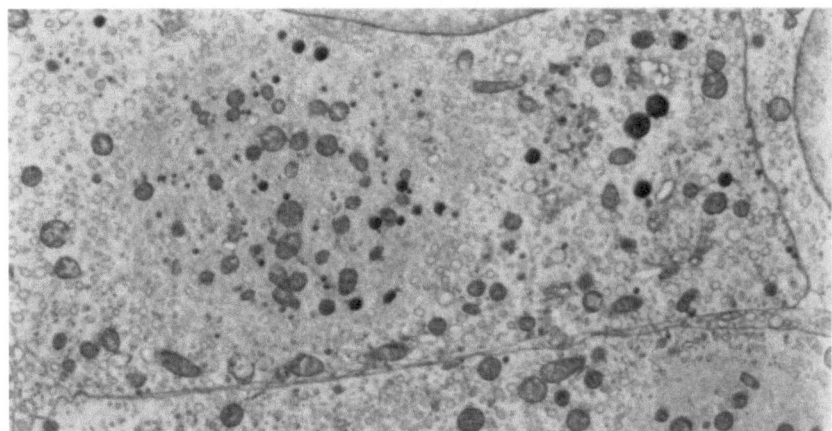

Fig. 60. Endocrine inactive pituitary adenoma: Spherical aggregation of intracytoplasmatic fibrils enclosing mitochondria, vesicles, and secretory granules producing a picture similar to that found in cases with acromegaly (Figs. 17, 20). Case 2/71, osmium, × 7,600

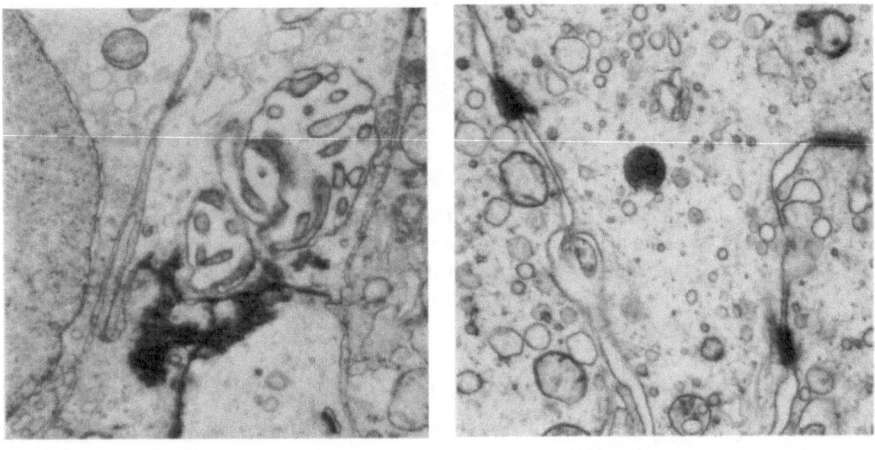

Fig. 61   Fig. 62

Fig. 61. Endocrine inactive pituitary adenoma: Formation of abortive follicle by cell processes lacking secretory granules. Case 46/72, osmium, × 15,600

Fig. 62. Endocrine inactive pituitary adenoma: Desmosomes between agranular cells in case with extensive follicle formation. Case 64/72, osmium, × 18,200

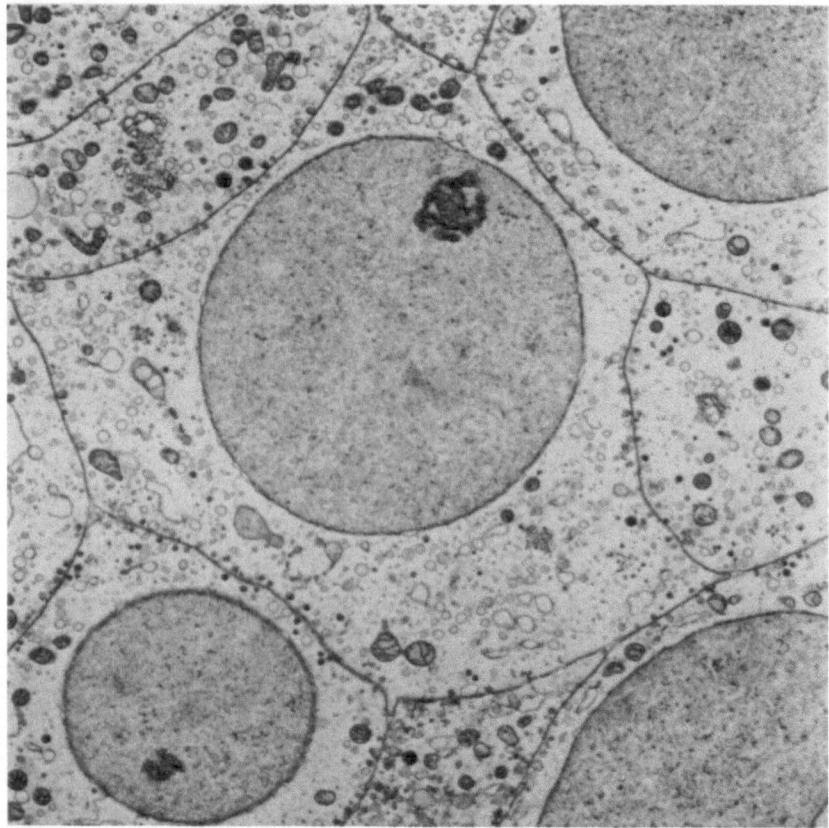

Fig. 63. Endocrine inactive pituitary adenoma: Cells with low content of organelles consisting mainly of empty vesicles, dense core vesicles closely apposed to the cell membrane, mitochondria, and Golgi cisterns. Case 11/71, osmium, ×7,000

dispersed among them. Similar findings have been described in two of 18 chromophobe adenomas in another series (Fukuda, 1973). This type of adenoma is easily differentiated from the ACTH producing tumor of Bergland and Torack (1969a) since the secretory cells themselves in the latter situation are engaged in the formation of the follicles. There are no clinical features in our own two cases which could be used for separation from the remaining large group of cases with endocrine inactive adenomas.

The remaining 32 cases of our series do not show any special features allowing a possible functional classification in spite of the fact that the ultrastructural examination demonstrates signs of active secretion. The

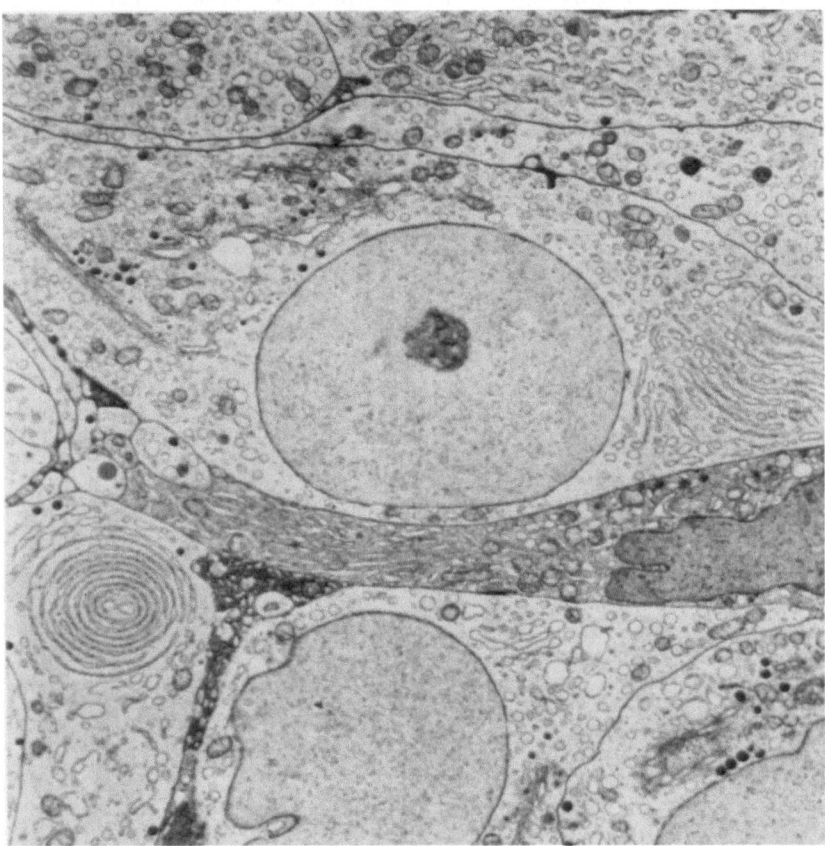

Fig. 64. Endocrine inactive pituitary adenoma: Tumor consisting of cells containing extremely well developed RER with "nebenkern" formation and numerous Golgi cisterns. The dark cell with pycnotic nucleus is probably undergoing necrobiotic changes. Case 6/73, osmium, ×5,300

cells are usually polygonal and in close juxtaposition (Figs. 63 and 64). The nuclei are round or oval in 20 and polymorphic in 12 cases. The organelle content is quite low (Fig. 63) in some adenomas whereas others contain an abundance of different organelles (Fig. 64). The first type contains some vesicles, mitochondria, and secretory granules of moderate electron density which are mainly lined up along the cell membrane. Some rare examples show nearly no granules at all. Golgi cisterns are infrequent and of limited dimensions. The RER is inconspicuous. The second type contains numerous Golgi saccules and a well developed RER which occasionally forms circular arrays designated as "nebenkern" (Fig. 64). One case even demonstrated the presence of annulate lamellae

(Fig. 65). Both signs suggest increased protein synthesis. The formation and secretion of electron dense secretory granules can be observed in all stages. Tumor forms intermediate between the two examples described exist. Six cases demonstrate numerous lysosomes engaged in phagocytosis and digestion of the secretory granules (Fig. 66). This observation

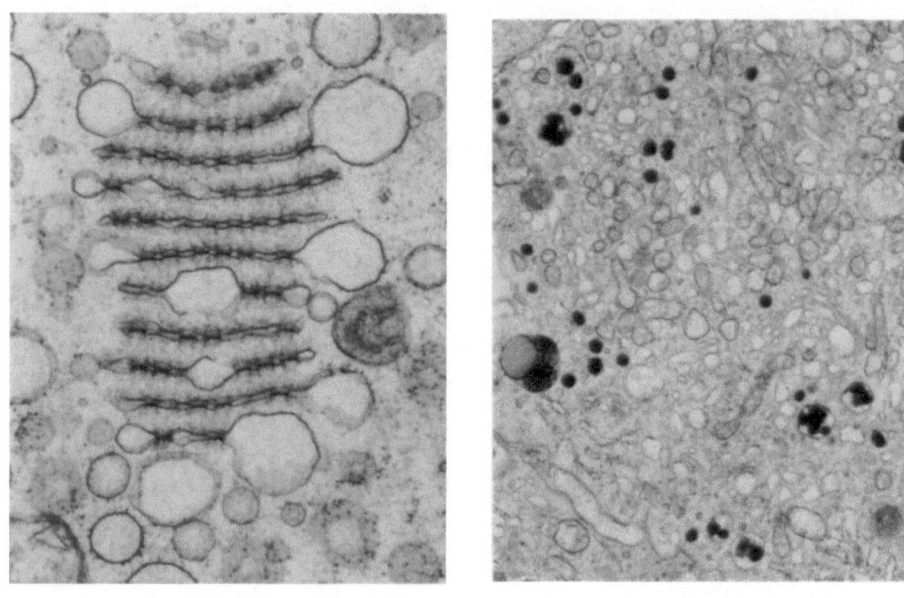

Fig. 65   Fig. 66

Fig. 65. Endocrine inactive pituitary adenoma: Formation of annulate lamellae in conjunction with cisterns of dilatated RER. Case 62/73, osmium, × 23,800

Fig. 66. Endocrine inactive pituitary adenoma: Tumor cell containing numerous lysosomes engaged in crinophagy and formation of lipid bodies. Case 6/71, osmium, × 11,800

can explain the lack of endocrinological symptoms: it may be that no active hormone reaches the blood circulation. Further investigations with immunohistochemical methods will be necessary to get a clearer insight into the nature of the synthesized material in these adenomas.

In most cases the blood vessels of endocrine inactive adenomas show the same ultrastructural findings as in acromegaly (see page 46). We have one exception: a case with undulating tubular structures in the perinuclear cistern and in the cisterns of the RER of the endothelial cells. In addition the same case demonstrates multilayered basal membranes with an increased thickness. No penetration of adenoma cells through the capillary walls have been observed.—The most striking contrast with normal pituitary capillaries is the relative paucity of endothelial fenestrae and the frequency of Weibel-Palade bodies (Weibel and Palade, 1964) in the tumors accompanied by a widened perivascular space as noted by others (Hirano *et al.*, 1972).

6. Malignant Pituitary Tumors

Adenohypophysial tumors usually grow in an expansive manner. The primary effects of tumors without positive endocrinological symptoms result from compression of the normal pituitary gland or nearby neuronal structures—particularly the optic chiasm and optic nerves. Expansive growth can give rise to extremely large tumors that compress the third ventricle or erode the sphenoid bone. There is a minority of tumors with locally invasive growth extending beyond the dural capsule into the cavernous sinus, middle cranial fossa, temporal lobe, diencephalon, clivus, sphenoid sinus, and epipharynx. A small number of tumors may metastasize to the subarachnoid space remote from the primary lesion, to extracranial organs via the blood circulation, or to both (Table 13).

Many clinicians and some pathologists have considered that invasiveness indicates malignancy (Jefferson, 1954; Kraus 1945; Newton et al., 1962) whereas Bailey (1932) stated that invasion into neighbouring structures is not indicative of malignancy. According to widely accepted criteria the only tumors with proven malignancy are those with distant metastases. But even in this group considerable variation in biological behaviour and the histological picture has been noted. Despite considerable work done by many authors, there is still no definite agreement as to what constitutes a carcinoma of the pituitary gland. We will classify both invasive and metastasizing tumors as "malignant".

Recurrences of malignant tumors manifested by the presence of metastases may appear after some weeks (Braun and Tzonos, 1965) or after several years (Solitaire and Jatlow, 1967) in spite of the same histological picture. Relative insensitivity to X-ray treatment is common among many metastasizing and invasive pituitary tumors (Ennuyer and Cheguillaume, 1958; Feiring et al., 1953; Jefferson, 1954; Wise et al., 1955). Martins and coauthors (1965) have shown that at least some invasive tumors can be cured by combined treatment with surgery and radiotherapy.—Since signs of malignancy can be detected only late in the course of the disease, the question has been raised whether X-irradiation might have a carcinogenic effect in pre-existing adenomas (Solitaire and Jatlow, 1967). This was based on the observation of four patients with malignant cranial neoplasms (anaplastic carcinoma presumably arising in a paranasal sinus or the middle ear, hemangioendothelioma, and two fibrosarcomas) found in a series of 75 cases previously treated with radiation therapy for acromegaly (Goldberg et al., 1963). A possible relationship has been denied by other authors (Svien and Colby, 1967) or has been judged as very uncommon (Newton et al., 1962).

From the literature we have collected 25 cases in which metastases

Table 13. *Endocrine Function and Sites of Metastases of Malignant Pituitary Tumors*

Author(s)	Type of endo-crinological syndrome	Sites of metastases	Type of metastatic spreading
Braun and Tzonos, 1965	inactive	frontal lobe, dura	S
Cagnetto, 1904	acromegaly	spine	S
Cairns and Russell, 1931	inactive	spine	S
Epstein et al., 1964	inactive	cauda equina	S
Fasske, 1958	inactive	base of brain	S
Feiring et al., 1953	Cushing	anterior cranial fossa	S
Gullotta and Klein, 1973	inactive	brachium conjunct.	S
Kontchakowa, 1936	acromegaly	pedunculus cerebri, tuber cinereum	S
Madonick et al., 1963	inactive	frontal lobe, spine	S
Newton et al., 1962	acromegaly, galactorrhea	hippocampus	S
Smoler, 1909	inactive	cerebellum	S
Solitaire and Jatlow, 1967	inactive	frontal lobe	S
Cohen and Dibble, 1936	Cushing	liver	H
Dott et al., 1925; Henderson, 1939	inactive	liver	H
Frobes, 1947	Cushing	liver	H
Geroulanos, 1969	inactive	liver, bone	H
Gilmour, 1932	inactive	liver, kidney, bladder uterus, vagina, lymph nodes	H
Köhlmeier, 1944	inactive	liver	H
McLean, 1936	inactive	"abdominal organs" (2 cases)	H
Moberg, 1959	inactive	heart	H
Scholz et al., 1962	inactive	cervical lymph nodes	H
Sheldon et al., 1954	Cushing	liver	H
Graf et al., 1962	inactive	frontal lobe, liver, lung	S, H
Salassa et al., 1959	Cushing	spinal, liver	S, H

S: subarachnoid metastases; H: hematogenous metastases.

were proven either at autopsy or by surgery (Table 13). There were 17 tumors either with hypopituitarism or without signs of endocrine activity, five cases with Cushing's syndrome, and three cases with acromegaly (one combined with galactorrhea). The large number of corticotrophic tumors is noteworthy if the relative rarity of this syndrome is kept in mind.—Eleven tumors metastasised through the blood stream, twelve via the subarachnoid space, and two through both mechanisms. Most hematogenous metastases were localized in the liver (8 cases). The lung was affected only once (Graf *et al.*, 1962) in spite of the fact that the tumor has to pass the pulmonary filter before reaching the liver.

A careful search for other possible primary cancers has to be made in every case of suspected metastatic pituitary tumor. There are reports indicating that the pituitary gland itself is harboring metastases in 0.14–26.6% of all cancer patient autopsies (Abrams *et al.*, 1950; Delarue *et al.*, 1964; Hägerstrand and Schönebeck, 1969; Hauck *et al.*, 1970; Kovacs, 1973; Roessmann *et al.*, 1970; Rose and Mennig, 1969; Simonds, 1914; Walther, 1948; Wyeth, 1934). Even a case of a metastasis to an eosinophilic pituitary adenoma has been reported (Richardson and Katayama, 1971). The most frequent site of the primary neoplasm is the mammary gland.

Most histological studies of metastatic pituitary tumors as well as invasive adenomas have demonstrated an abnormal cellular pattern when compared to the average pituitary adenoma (Bailey and Cutler, 1940; Dott *et al.*, 1925; Feiring *et al.*, 1953; Frazier, 1930; Henderson, 1939; Jefferson, 1954; Kernohan and Sayre, 1956; King, 1951; Martins *et al.*, 1965; Wise *et al.*, 1955). Polymorphism of cells and nuclei, multiple nuclei, absence of stainable granules, increased number of mitoses, and abnormal mitotic figures have been described as characterizing invasive and metastasizing pituitary tumors. Sarcomatous changes have been noted (Moberg, 1959). The criteria enumerated characterize a malignant tumor only if occurring together since polymorphism, multinucleation, and presence of mitoses can be observed in strictly localized benign pituitary adenomas (Bailey and Cushing, 1928; Brion and Fanjoux, 1958, Newton *et al.*, 1962; Robert, 1973). Not even the absence of stainable granules can be used as a single criterion since metastasizing eosinophilic and basophilic metastatic tumors have been reported (Cagnetto, 1904; Cohen and Dible, 1936; Graf *et al.*, 1962; Jefferson, 1954; Sheldon *et al.*, 1954). Some tumors with distant metastases demonstrated a very regular structure on histologic examination (Frobes, 1947; Madonick *et al.*, 1963; Scholz *et al.*, 1962). These observations show that histology often is not able to clarify the biological behaviour of a pituitary tumor.

Luse (1961, 1962) was convinced that pronounced polymorphism of nuclei on ultrastructural examination was characteristic of malignant pituitary tumors. The cytoplasm of her cases did not show any particular features. This view was opposed by Brucher and coworkers (1970) who considered that polymorphism of nuclei was not sufficient evidence of an advanced degree of anaplasia indicating a malignant pituitary tumor. These authors assumed that loss of cytoplasmic differentiation as well as nuclear irregularities and changes in the nuclear—cytoplasmic ratio were important criteria. They also thought that the loss of granule production might be an important clue. This latter suggestion was not supported by the results of ultrastructural examination of formalin-fixed tissue taken from a metastatic pituitary tumor without signs of endocrine activity (Gullotta and Klein, 1973). The cells contained an abundance of electron-dense granules in spite of an unsatisfactory tissue preservation.

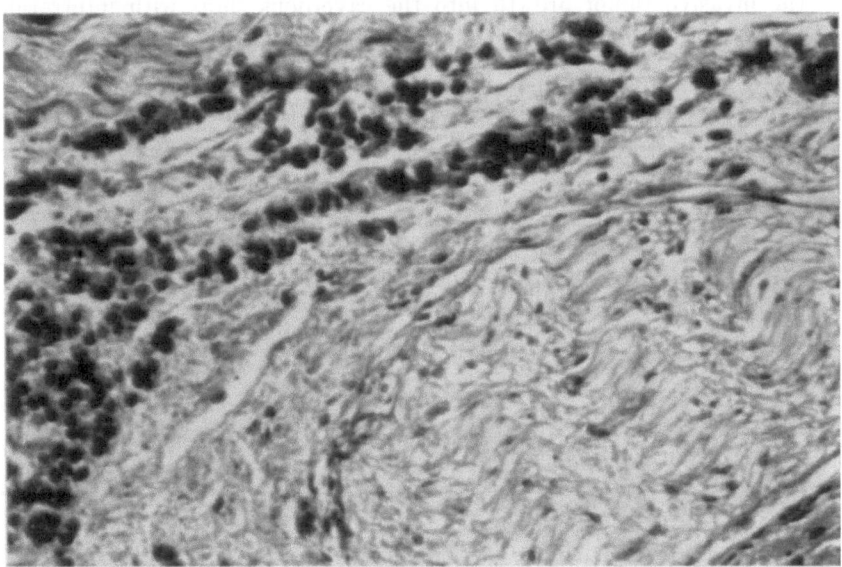

Fig. 67. Invasive pituitary adenoma with Forbes-Albright syndrome: Adenoma cells invading cavernous sinus between bundles of trigeminal nerve fibres. Autopsy material, light micrograph, formalin fixation, H & E, ×330

Our own material contains seven biopsies from five patients with locally invasive tumors. There were two cases without endocrine activity, one 14 year old boy with gigantism secondary to a HGH producing tumor, one patient with Nelson's syndrome, and one patient with Forbes-Albright syndrome. All patients except one had shown clinical signs of cavernous sinus invasion.—Two patients died. No autopsy was obtained from the case with gigantism, but the other showed invasive growth. This latter patient had a Forbes-Albright syndrome (see also page 51) with secondary amenorrhea and galactorrhea since the age of 20 years. She was operated upon for the first time at the age of 28 years and received a course of postoperative X-ray therapy (5,000 rads local dose). She started to suffer from recurrent deterioration of vision with ultimate blindness two years after irradiation. Progressive diabetes insipidus, organic psychosyndrome, and voracious appetite were observed later during the course of the disease. She was reoperated upon twice (one transsphenoidal, one transfrontal approach) because of suspected regrowth. Surgery demonstrated local adhesions and scar tissue invaded by the tumor. There was no space occupying lesion on either occasion. The patient died at the age of 31 years with severe electrolyte disturbances.—The histological examination of autopsy material demonstrated the invasive tumor growth into the cavernous sinus with infiltration between the branches of the fifth cranial nerve (Fig. 67). The tumor

Table 14. *Clinical Findings in Five Cases with Invasive Pituitary Adenomas*

Case number	Endocrine syndrome	Cranial nerve lesions	Survival since first symptoms (years)	Result
48/73	inactive	III, V_1, V_2, V_{motor}	$2\frac{1}{2}$	L
42/73	inactive	III, V_1, V_2	$3\frac{1}{2}$	L
15/71	gigantism	II, III	$5\frac{1}{2}$	D_1
16/71	Nelson	III, (IV)	7	L
35/73	Forbes-Albright	II (radiation damage)	$11\frac{1}{2}$	D_2

Explanation: L living;
D_1 dead, cause unknown, no autopsy;
D_2 dead, radiation necrosis of hypothalamus.

cells contained erythrosine positive granules. There was neither cellular anaplasia nor an increased number of mitoses, multinucleation, or nuclear pleomorphism present. The hypothalamus showed extensive areas of necrosis with focal calcifications, fibrosis and hyalinosis of the small blood vessels, and reactive gliosis. These changes are known to be typical for irradiation damage of the brain in man (Blackwood *et al.*, 1963; Crompton and Layton, 1961; Krayenbühl and Rüttner, 1973; Lampert and Davis, 1964; Pennybaker and Russell, 1948; Rubinstein, 1972; Zülch, 1960, 1969). Careful histological examination demonstrated no invasion into the optic nerves or the brain.

The clinical findings in our cases, recorded in Table 14, demonstrate the long course in our patients. The oculomotor nerve usually was affected first, later the trigeminal nerve was occasionally involved. We have not yet seen damage to the fourth cranial nerve. The latter nerves were rarely affected in the cases collected by Jefferson (1954). Surgical decompression was followed in all cases by only a partial improvement

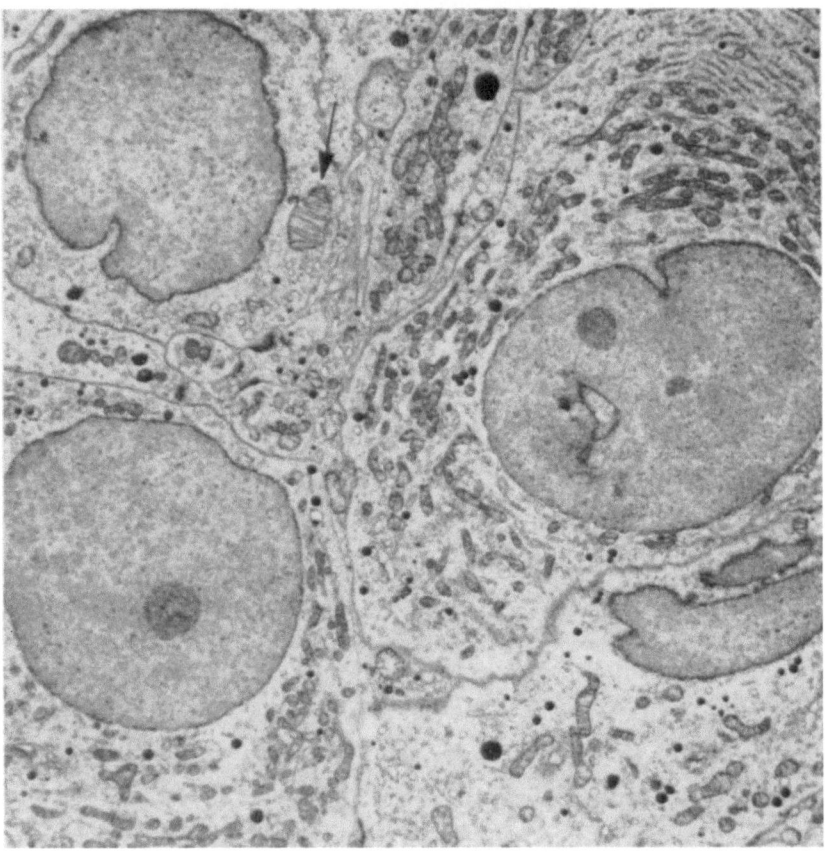

Fig. 68. Invasive pituitary adenoma without signs of endocrine activity: Densely arranged cells demonstrating nuclear polymorphism and accumulation of numerous cytoplasmic organelles. One giant mitochondrion (arrow) and a fair number of secretory granules can be seen. Case 48/73, osmium, × 5,500

in the nerve function; in most cases this improvement lasted only a few months. Only the patient with Nelson's syndrome showed a restoration of abducens function, and this has persisted for 3 years. The oculomotor paresis did not change. Radiotherapy did not show any beneficial effect in our cases.

In four of our cases the histological examination of the biopsies shows ordinary adenoma tissue without increased numbers of mitoses or cellular or nuclear polymorphism. An increased number of mitoses with moderate polymorphism of nuclei are present in only one case without signs of endocrine activity (case 42/73). The cells of the case with

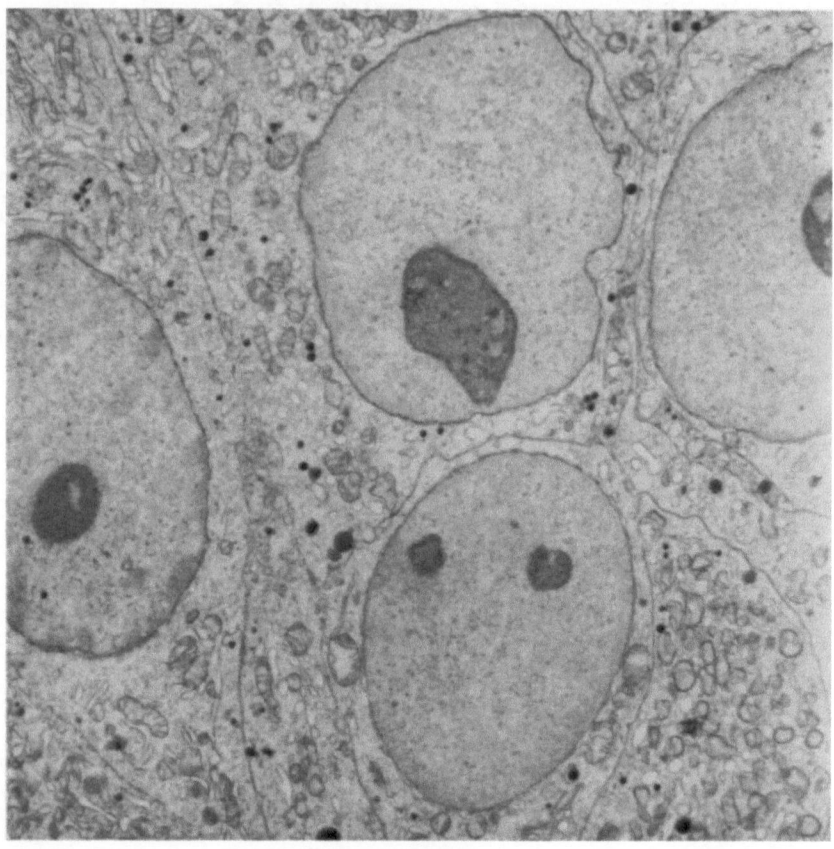

Fig. 69. Invasive pituitary adenoma without signs of endocrine activity:
Presence of multiple and abnormally large nucleoli. Case 48/73, osmium,
× 7,000

gigantism contain eosinophilic granules and those of the case with Forbes-
Albright syndrome, erythrosinophilic granules.

The results of electron microscopy confirm the findings of conventional histology. There is no evidence of cellular anaplasia present. The
tumor cells usually are arranged in a compact pattern (Figs. 68, 69, and
70). Small, empty intercellular spaces are present only in the case with
gigantism. The cells are usually polygonal and of uniform size. No
multinuclear cells can be observed. The nuclei generally are round or
oval and only occasionally demonstrate some polymorphism (Fig. 68).
The nucleoli are often multiple or abnormally large (Fig. 69). The
nuclear-cytoplasmic ratio does not seem to be different from noninvasive
adenomas. The cytoplasm contains a large number of organelles with

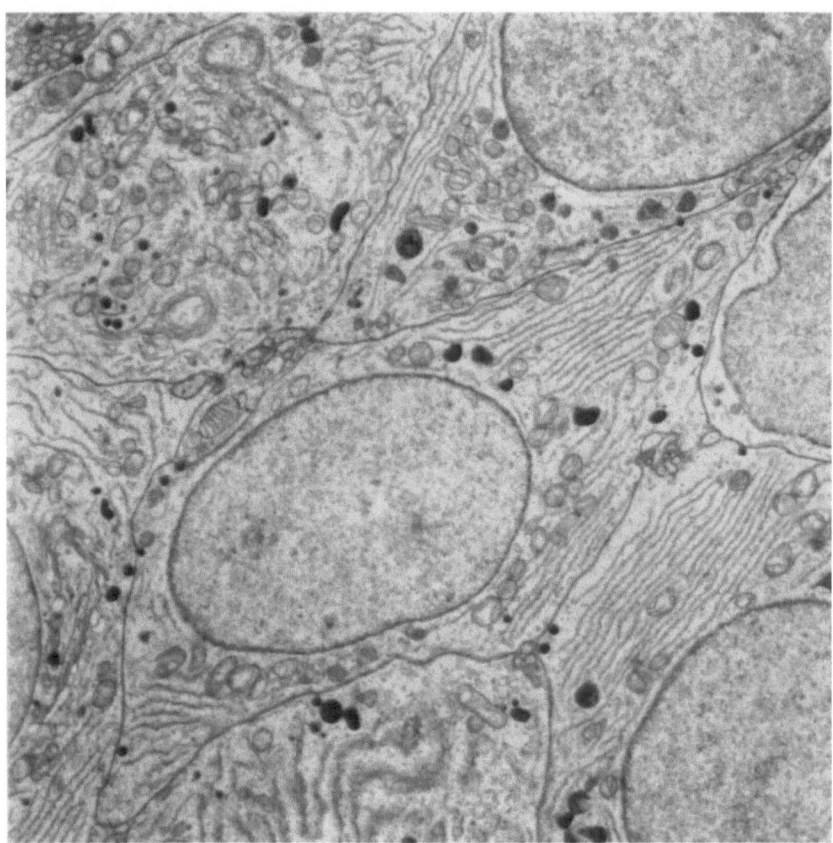

Fig. 70. Invasive pituitary adenoma without signs of endocrine activity: Cytoplasm containing extremely well developed RER, multiple, irregularly arranged Golgi cisterns (upper left corner), and numerous large and deformed secretory granules. Case 42/73, osmium, × 8,200

numerous mitochondria and a RER which is occasionally quite elaborate (Fig. 70). The Golgi cisterns seem to be somewhat more irregular than usual. All five tumors of this series contain numerous secretory granules. Their electron density varies from case to case but is usually high as demonstrated by the adenoma producing the amenorrhea-galactorrhea syndrome (Fig. 71). One case without signs of endocrine activity demonstrates unusually polymorphic granules (Fig. 70).

The examination of tumor cells invading intrasellar scar tissue (case 35/73) shows that the strands of tumor cells are separated from the collagenous fiber accumulations by seemingly uninterrupted basal membranes (Fig. 71). This observation casts some doubt on the assumption

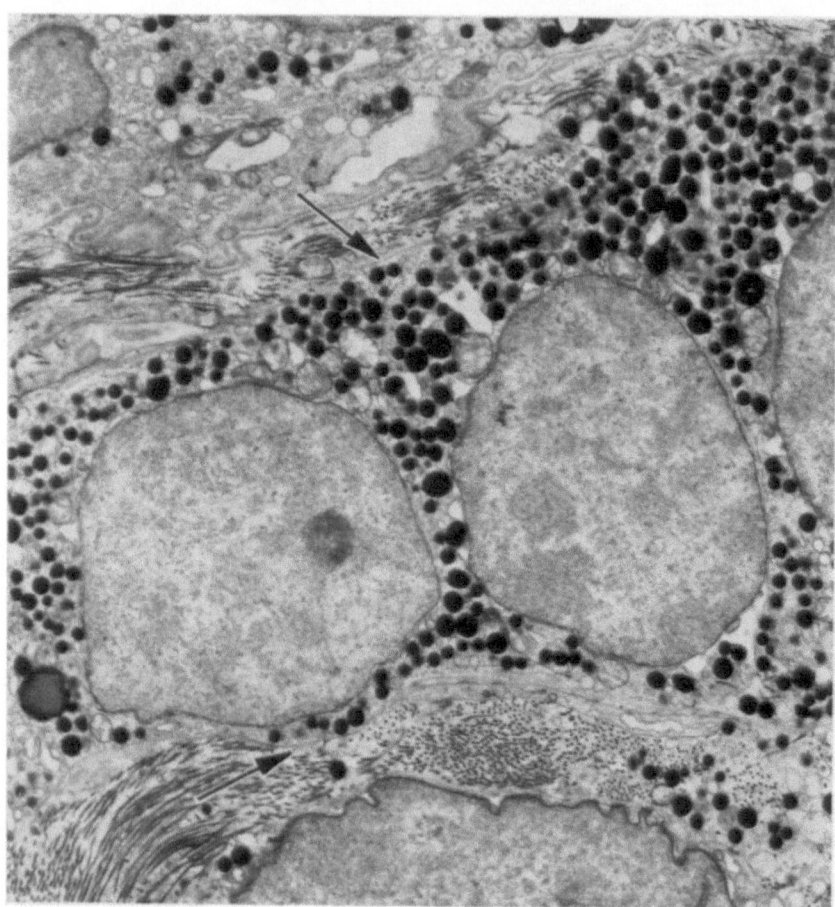

Fig. 71. Invasive pituitary adenoma with Forbes-Albright syndrome: Heavily granulated epithelial cells are separated from surrounding collagen fibrils by continuous basal membranes (arrows).   Case 35/73, osmium, × 8,200

that invasive pituitary adenomas have to be classified as malignant.— The ultrastructure of capillaries in our five cases does not differ from the noninvasive adenomas. No disruption of basal membranes or invasions of tumor cells have been observed.

The ultrastructure of invasive pituitary tumors therefore does not show any clear cut differences when compared with noninvasive adenomas. There are only minor differences such as the presence of multiple or enlarged nucleoli. There are no signs of anaplasia. In some cases the secretory activity is maintained as demonstrated by electron microscopy or clinical symptoms. The further examination of pituitary carcinomas with distant metastases may show if significant differences exist in comparison with pituitary adenomas. But this may be unlikely since the single case examination reported to date (Gullotta and Klein, 1973) contained a large number of secretory granules. A definite decision concerning the growth characteristics of a given pituitary tumor probably cannot be made with microscopic techniques alone.

7. Craniopharyngiomas

Craniopharyngiomas represent the second most frequent tumor of the intra- and suprasellar region in man. They account for 2–3% of all intracranial tumors (Svolos, 1969: 1.94%; Zülch, 1956: 2.7%; Russell and Rubinstein, 1971: 3%). Our own series contains 92 pituitary adenomas and 16 craniopharyngiomas (17%) whose ultrastructure has been examined. The youngest patient was 3; the oldest 55 years old. Eight patients were in the first decade of life, 4 in the second, and 4 in the third, fourth and fifth. The age distribution shows the same predominance of patients in the first two decades of life as seen in other series (Bailey et al., 1939; Cushing, 1932b; Frazier and Alpers, 1931; Gordy et al., 1949; Love and Marshall, 1950; Northfield, 1957) although this shift is somewhat more pronounced in our material. There were 8 male and 8 female patients. The tumors were usually located in the suprasellar region. They frequently showed intrasellar, retrosellar, and parasellar extensions. One cystic craniopharyngioma showed an exclusively intrasellar location (no. 11/73). Two had grown into the third ventricle and were therefore removed on a transventricular approach.

Three or four different tissue components are found in craniopharyngiomas as reported in the first description by Erdheim (1904). The four elements are epithelium, collagenous connective tissue, capillaries and astroglia. They always are strictly separated from each other by uninterrupted basal membranes (Landolt, 1972). The architecture of the different tumors shows a considerable degree of variation, but all types are derived from the same basic structure (Fig. 72). The variations are caused by differing proliferative tendencies of the epithelium and the stroma (del Vivo et al., 1962).

The basic structure is represented by a *simple cyst* lined by a wall of connective tissue and a multilayered squamous epithelium which does not proliferate and even shows regressive changes. The second group shows a proliferative tendency of the epithelium lining the cystic cavity. The proliferation can be localized mainly in the squamous layer or in the basal layer. In the former the epithelium forms papillary structures in the cyst cavity (*papillary cyst*). In the latter, characterized by an even greater proliferation of the epithelium the basocellular growth predominates (*basocellular type*). Three types of basocellular evolution can be differentiated: The *cylindromatous type* is characterized by a progressive liquefication of the connective tissue islands surrounded by the epithelial masses. The final stage of this regression shows a complete disappearance of the connective tissue giving way to empty spaces. The basal membrane therefore delineates a circumscribed cavity. The *adamantinomatous type* shows alterations similar to those of the adamantinoma: stellate reticu-

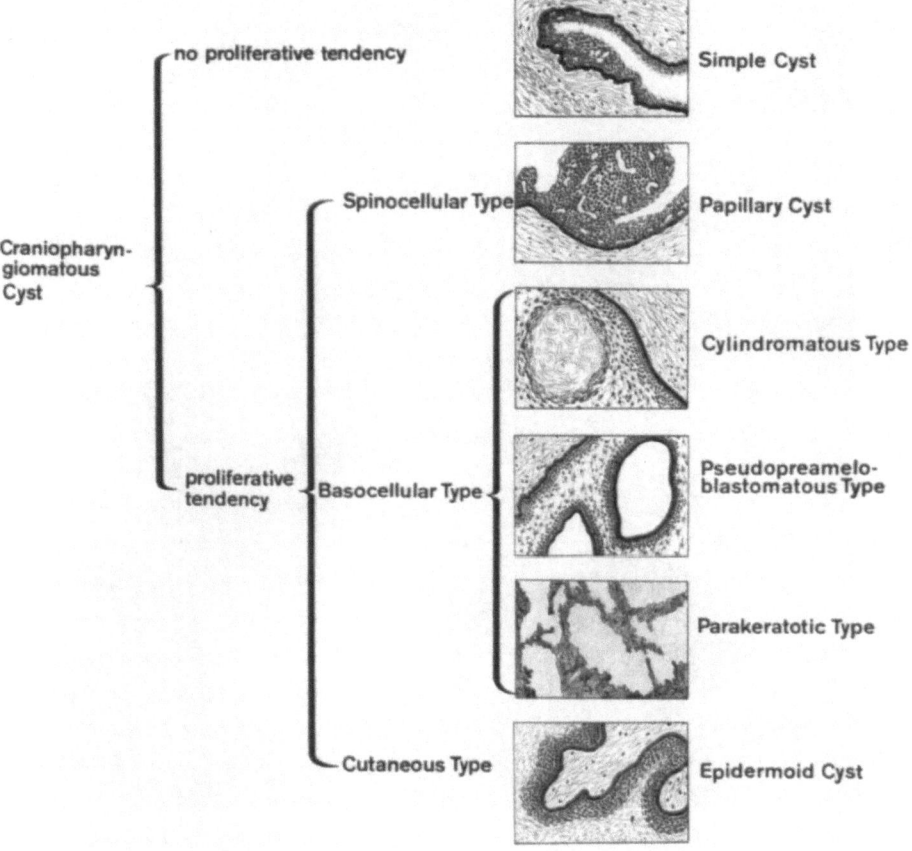

no proliferative tendency — Simple Cyst

Spinocellular Type — Papillary Cyst

Craniopharyn-
giomatous
Cyst

Cylindromatous Type

proliferative tendency — Basocellular Type — Pseudopreamelo-blastomatous Type

Parakeratotic Type

Cutaneous Type — Epidermoid Cyst

Fig. 72. Diagramatic representation of the histogenic relations of the different types of craniopharyngiomatous cysts according to del Vivo *et al.* (1962). For further explanation see text

lum resembling the enamel organ with focal squamous transformation and defective keratinization (Anderson, 1953; Lichtenstein, 1972). The third type presents large areas of *parakeratotic transformation* with more or less complete disappearance of viable epithelial cells similar to Malherbe's epithelioma (Pinkus and Mehregan, 1973). Therefore, according to this interpretation the *epidermoid cysts* of the sella region belong to the craniopharyngiomas. Their peculiar evolution shows the morphological aspects of the skin in different variations.

This analysis suggests that each craniopharyngioma starts from a squamous epithelium cyst originating from the remnants of the hypophysial duct. According to this view the tumors derived from these

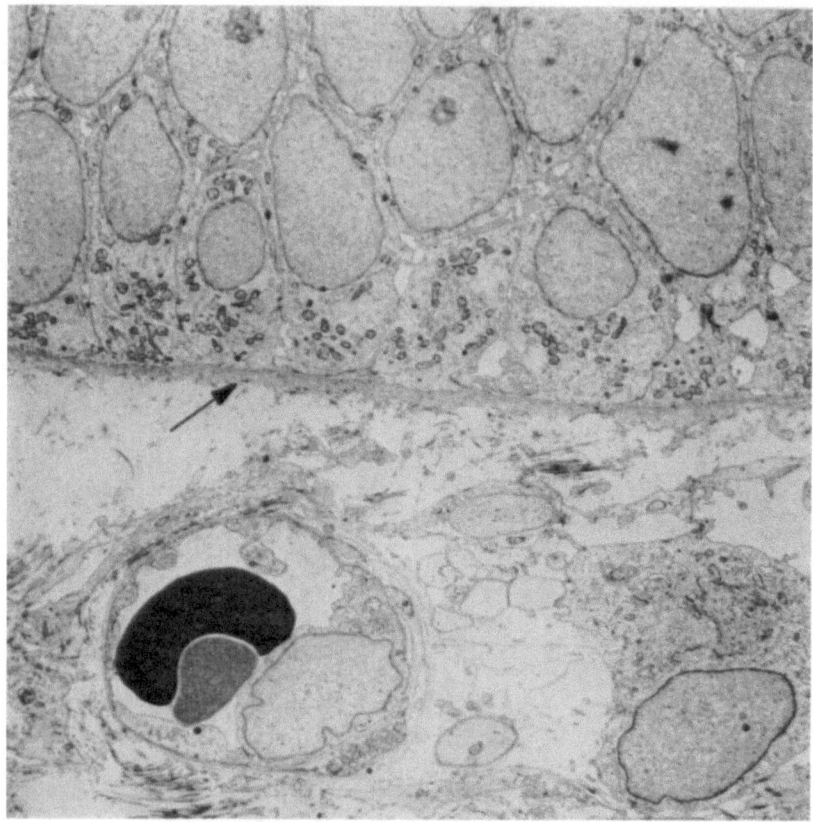

Fig. 73. Craniopharyngioma: Basal epithelial layer (upper part of micrograph) consisting of densely apposed, elongated cells separated by basal membrane (arrow) from loose stroma containing capillary, fibroblasts and collagen fibrils. Case 37/72, osmium, × 3,700

cysts are hamartomas. The different histological forms are only the consequence of successive changes in evolution. It seems likely that the surrounding tissues (stroma) which come into contact with the epithelial cyst play an important role in the development of the primary malformation.

The electron microscope allows excellent insight into the changes occurring in the different tissue components. These changes are represented by various processes of differentiation and degeneration as well as secondary processes, *e.g.*, calcification. The degree of differentiation as well as degeneration varies from tumor to tumor and sometimes even from one section in one tumor to an adjacent one. Therefore the architecture of a tumor can be evaluated better in survey micrographs ob-

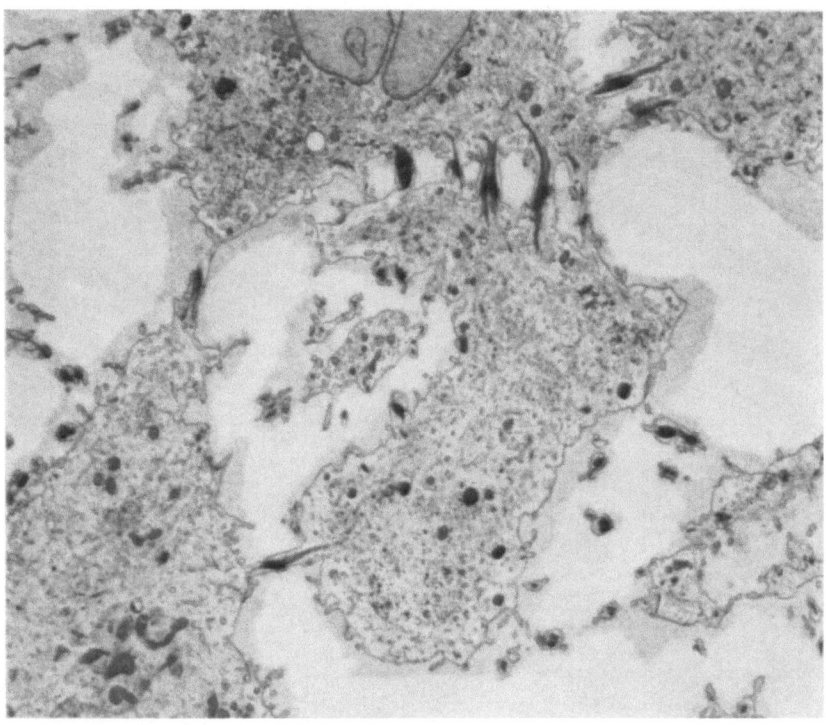

Fig. 74. Craniopharyngioma: Central part of epithelial component consisting of stellate cells with slender processes and large intercellular space with flocular material condensed along cell surfaces. The cells contain mitochondria, lipid bodies, and numerous fibrils forming densely packed bundles in the cell processes. Case 27/71, osmium, × 5,600

tained with the light microscope whereas the examination of electron microscopic pictures allows the evaluation of the processes involved.

Results of the electron microscopic examination of craniopharyngiomas have been reported by Foncin (1971), Ghatak et al. (1971), Hossmann and Wechsler (1967), Landolt (1972, 1974b), Luse (1962), Nyström (1973), and Poon et al. (1971). The epithelial components of the tumors are always surrounded by a continuous basal membrane which separates them from the stroma (Fig. 73). Despite variations in size, shape, and arrangement, the fine structure of the epithelial cells shows certain characteristic features such as the presence of desmosomes and tonofilaments. These structures or their derivatives can be found in every type of epithelial differentiation. The polygonal or elongated cells are densely packed in the basal layers leaving only occasionally some intercellular space (Fig. 80). The nuclei occupy the largest part of the cell volume.

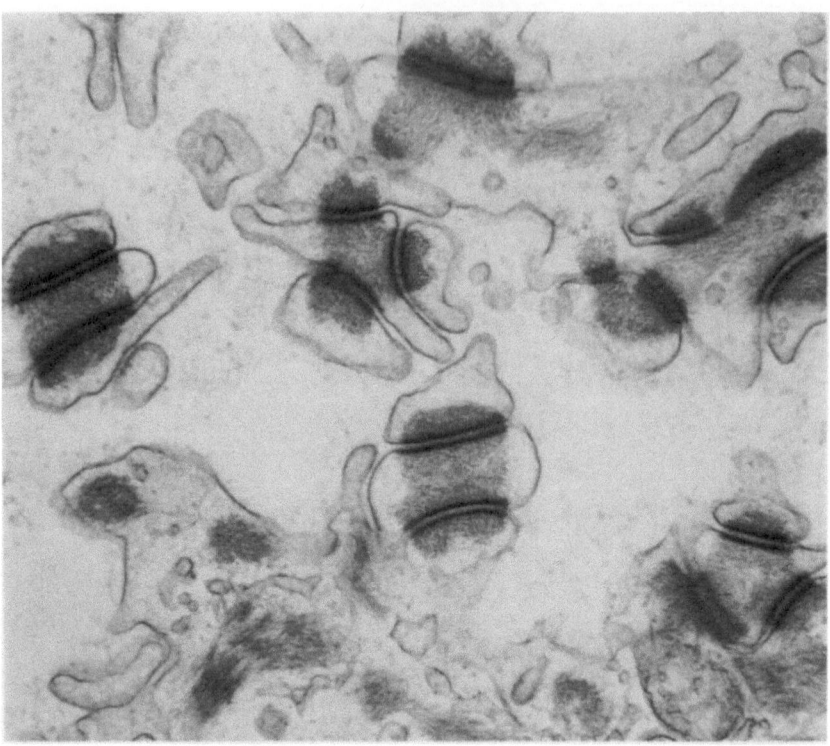

Fig. 75. Craniopharyngioma: High magnification micrograph of epithelial
cell processes attached to each other by desmosomes to which the tonofilaments are attached. Case 27/71, osmium, × 29,900

They are usually round or oval but can show deep indentations. The
nucleoli are prominent. In addition a variable number of cytoplasmic
organelles can be observed including mitochondria, numerous vesicles,
smooth and rough surfaced endoplasmic reticulum, lysosomes, and occasional lipoid inclusions. The cells are attached to each other by numerous
desmosomes and contain a loose network of tonofilaments measuring
5 mμ in diameter. They are sometimes arranged in loose bundles and
lie at random within the cytoplasm. Hemidesmosomes can be seen on the
basal surface of the cell strands (see Fig. 9 of Landolt, 1972).

The intercellular spaces enlarge more and more towards the center of
the epithelial masses causing the appearance of prickle cells (Fig. 74).
This transformation is caused by the continuing adhesion of the cells in
the region of the desmosomes. Slender cell processes pulled out (Fig. 75).
The structure of the desmosomes remains unchanged. The tonofilaments
form bundles of increasing density which stay in contact with the desmo-

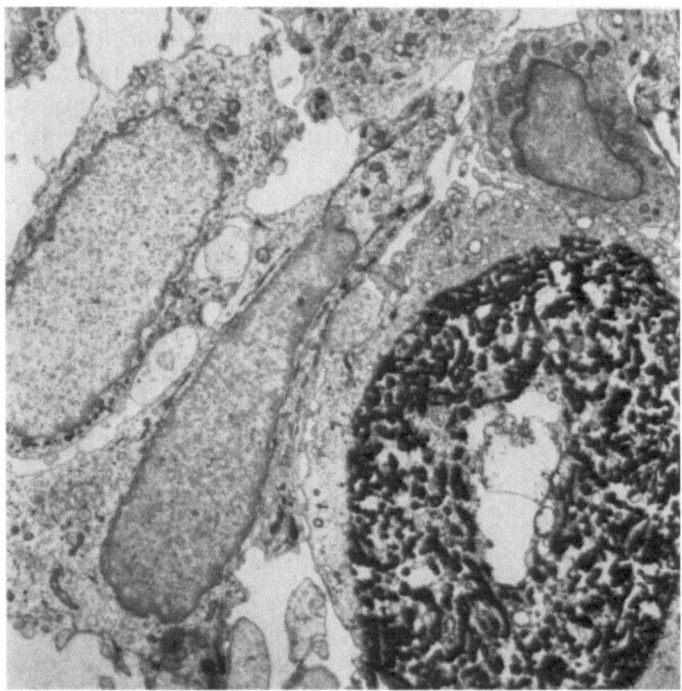

Fig. 76. Craniopharyngioma: Onionlike accumulation of epithelial cells with formation of parakeratotic center. The nucleus of the central cell is undergoing lysis. Its cytoplasm contains dense homogenous bundles of former tonofilaments. Case 12/73, osmium, ×4,500

somes. The character of the cells in the basal layers corresponds well to the stratum basale and spinosum of the normal epidermis (Brody, 1960; Parakkal and Alexander, 1972) although the intercellular space remains much smaller. The arrangement of the desmosomes and tonofilaments coincides in both tissues. The enamel organ of developing teeth contains the same cell type as the craniopharyngiomas. The extensive intercellular space shows the same dimensions in the stellate reticulum of the enamel organ (Elwood and Bernstein, 1968; Pannese, 1960).

Dense, onionlike accumulations of flattened epithelial cells are formed within the layer of basal cells or within the prickle cell reticulum (Fig. 76). Some accumulate lipoid droplets. The bundles of tonofilaments become larger in others. Dense homogenous granules are formed in contact with them (Fig. 77). The cell nuclei become pycnotic and the other cell organelles degenerate. The cell membrane disintegrates in certain regions but the desmosomes remain intact. Finally the cell is completely necrotic and the nucleus disappears leaving an empty space. The bundles of tonofilaments are turned into electron dense bands with a diameter of about 0.7 μ running in different directions through the former cell body (Fig. 78). Accumulations of fine, needlelike crystals can be seen in the necrotic cells. They easily can be identified as hydroxy apatite in selected area electron diffraction patterns (Landolt, 1972). This process

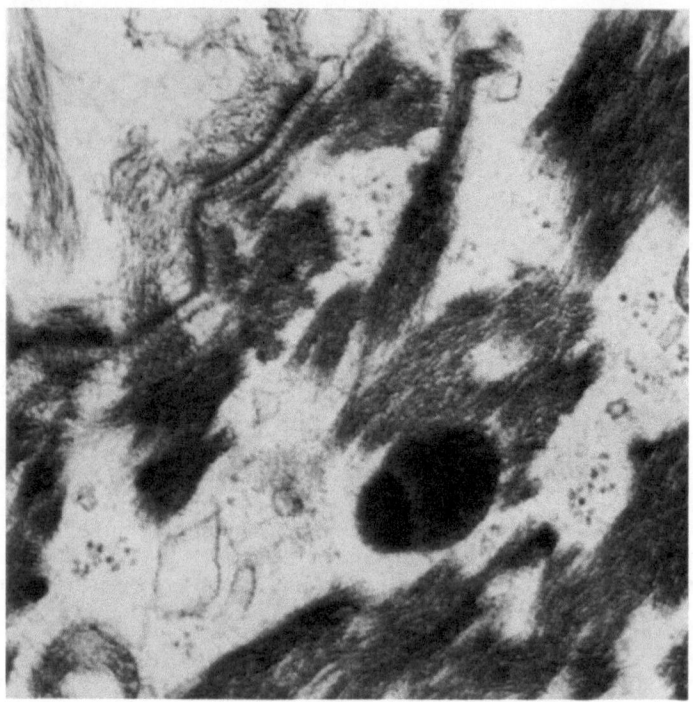

Fig. 77. Craniopharyngioma: Formation of dense keratohyalin granule in close contact with dense tonofilaments accumulation. Desmosome in upper left corner. Case 34/72, osmium, × 56,000

represents an abortive type of keratinization. The initial phases are indistinguishable from the normal (Brody, 1960; Odland and Reed, 1967; Parakkal and Alexander, 1972). Even small but typical keratohyalin granules can be recognized on the ultrastructural level (Fig. 76) although by light microscopy, these have been considered to be characteristically absent (Love and Marshall, 1950; Zülch, 1956). Our view is supported by the utrastructural findings of Ghatak et al. (1971). Additionally, cornification can be proven histochemically (Gon, 1965). The final step in keratinization, which is represented by the compact structure of the horny layer of skin, cannot be found in craniopharyngiomas. The keratin bundles remain unorganized leaving empty spaces which originally were occupied by different cell organelles and the nucleus. Only cellular debris remains. The type of abortive keratin formation described has to be called parakeratosis although major differences with the parakeratosis of psoriasis exist (Brody, 1962a, b). Calcifications existed in 2 of our 7

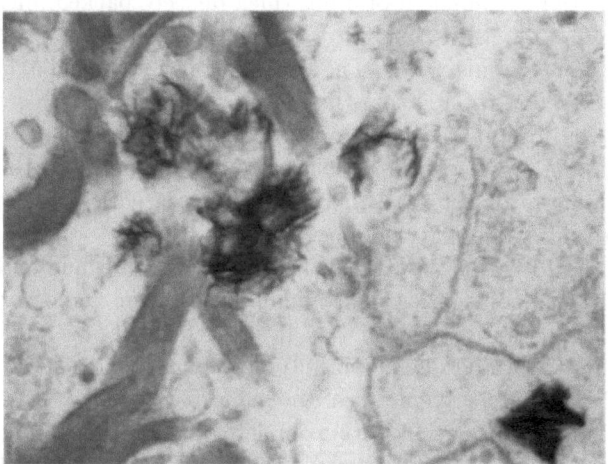

Fig. 78. Craniopharyngioma: Accumulation of needle-like hydroxyapatite crystals between homogenous bundles consisting of condensed former tonofilaments. Case 11/72, osmium, × 41,500

cases showing parakeratotic masses and have not been observed in the remaining 9 patients without them. This observation has been confirmed by light microscopy (Gon, 1965).

The ultrastructure of the epithelial components of craniopharyngiomas is similar to the calcifying odontogenic tumors (Anderson et al., 1969; Chaudhry et al., 1972; Mainwaring et al., 1971), the ameloblastomas (Mincer and McGinnis, 1972) and the adamantinomas (Spjut et al., 1971). The main constituent of all four tumors is a prismatic or stellate epithelial cell which shows bundles of tonofibrils and desmosomes. The primitive oral epithelium gives rise to several structures. At approximately the sixth week in utero oral epithelium proliferates and invaginates giving rise to the first tooth bud. At about the same time it evaginates as Rathke's pouch and contributes to the formation of the anterior pituitary gland. Between the seventh and the twelfth week in utero there is initiation of both major and minor salivary glands (Gorlin et al., 1961). The similarities in structure of craniopharyngiomas and odontogenic tumors therefore are not surprising. Consequently, the terms adamantinoma and ameloblastoma also have been used for craniopharyngiomas (Kerno-

han and Sayre, 1956). The relationship has been documented further by
the examination of rare craniopharyngiomas demonstrating tooth formation (Beck, 1883; Kalnins and Rossi, 1965; Pflüger and Schürmann,
1931; Seemayr *et al.*, 1972). The main difference between odontogenic
tumors and craniopharyngiomas is the extracellular and intracellular
deposition of amyloid producing a positive reaction with Congo red.
This material is composed of 5 mμ thick densely packed microfilaments
(Anderson *et al.*, 1969, Chaudhry *et al.*, 1972; Mainwaring *et al.*, 1971;
Mincer and McGinnis, 1972). The structure of the amyloid of odontogenic
tumors therefore differs from the amyloid associated with reticuloendo-
thelial cells (Shirahama and Cohen, 1967) even though both show the
positive Congo red reaction. The calcifications occur in this fibrillary
material in ameloblastomas whereas it is associated with the parakeratotic masses in craniopharyngiomas.

Biological relations continue to exist in the tooth bud and in craniopharyngiomas pointing to the common origin from the oral epithelium.
The enamel organ is sensitive to X-ray treatment (Cottier, 1966). Inten-
sive irradiation (no dosage reported) of a nevus on the check of a 2 year
old patient caused asymmetry of the mandible as well as severe disturbances of tooth formation with complete loss of the permanent teeth
(Zellner, 1959).—Craniopharyngiomas usually have been classified as
insensitive to irradiation or at least less sensitive to irradiation than the
surrounding nervous tissue. Consequently, radiotherapy usually is not
employed in the treatment of these tumors. However, increasing evidence has been presented that, despite its benign character, the tumor
can be treated successfully by transcutaneous X-radiation (Hoff and
Patterson, 1972; Kramer *et al.*, 1968; Svien and Colby, 1967) as well as
by intracystic application of yttrium-90 (Backlund, 1973). We recently
have presented the clinical and operative findings and the results of the
histological examination of tumor biopsies before and 4 years after
radiotherapy with a local dose of 4,000r in two patients (Landolt, 1974 b).
After radiation therapy the incompletely removed tumors consisted only
of shrunken scar tissue in which islands of parakeratotic masses and no
viable epithelial cells were embedded. A third tumor biopsy was examined with the electron microscope. The tissue consisted mainly of astrocytes with many Rosenthal fibres (see below) as well as large areas of
parakeratosis. There were only a few epithelial cells which had not yet
undergone the transformation into parakeratotic masses. All of them
were in an advanced stage of tonofibril accumulation.

The stroma of craniopharyngiomas consists of collagenous connective
tissue, blood vessels and, occasionally, fibrous glia. Collagenous tissue
can be detected in various amounts and in a different arrangement in
every case examined. Sometimes it forms only small strands. In other

instances it occupies large areas. Typical fibroblasts (Fig. 79) containing numerous mitochondria, Golgi structures, and saccular cisterns of the rough surfaced endoplasmic reticulum can be observed. The cells show slender processes and are surrounded by bundles of typical collagen fibrils. The tissue structure can be compact or can show focal areas of

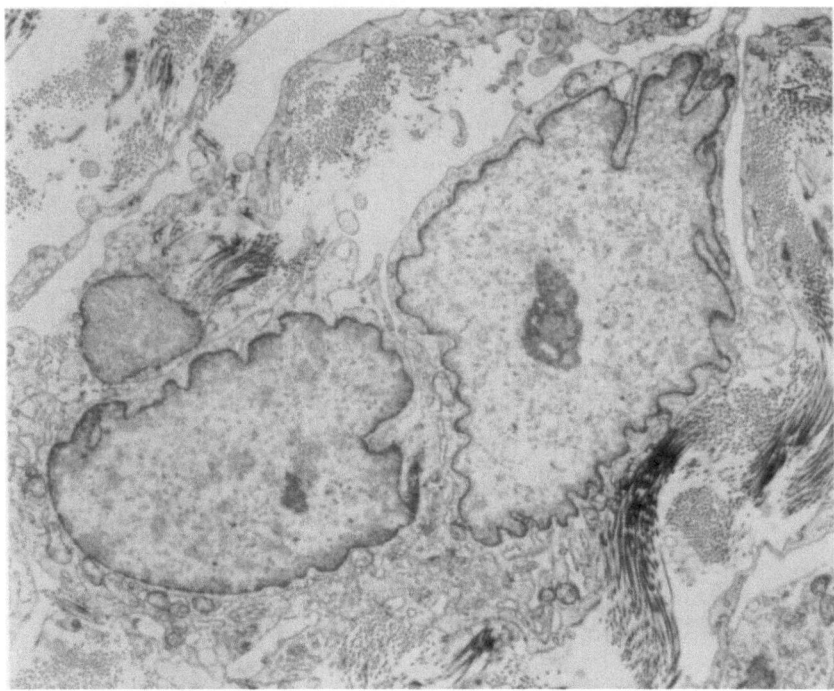

Fig. 79. Craniopharyngioma: Fibroblasts surrounded by loosely arranged collagen fibrils in tumor stroma. Case 37/73, osmium, × 7,100

rarefaction. This process of progressive disappearance of collagen fibrils and cellular components ultimately will lead to cystic cavities containing some floccular material (Fig. 80). These "cysts" are surrounded by a basal membrane and the basal layer of epithelial cells. Therefore they are situated outside of the epithelium and have to be classified as pseudocysts. This liquefication of the connective tissue leads to the cylindromatous type of craniopharyngiomas. Zülch (1971) described a secondary columnar transformation of the marginal epithelial lining of the cysts within the epithelial bands. This interpretation is incorrect because the cysts always are separated from the epithelial cells by an uninterrupted basal membrane and occasionally show few remaining collagen fibrils

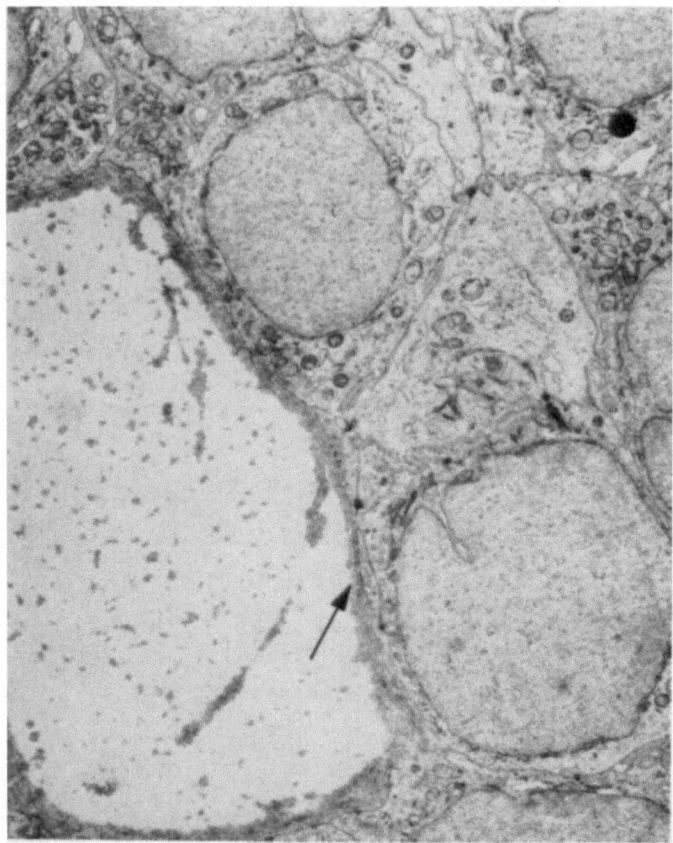

Fig. 80. Craniopharyngioma: Extraepithelial pseudocyst lined by basal membrane (arrow) and epithelial cells. The pseudocyst contains some floccular remnants of former stroma. Case 37/72, osmium, × 6,900

(see Fig. 95 of Zülch, 1971; and our Fig. 80). The extra-epithelial location of the cavities has been mentioned by various authors (del Vivo *et al.*, 1962; Russell and Rubinstein, 1971; Thibout, 1947). Intracytoplasmic lipid accumulation and necrosis of fibroblasts can be observed in some tumor specimen.

Five of the 16 craniopharyngiomas examined contain large areas occupied by astrocytes as part of the stroma. Some young astrocytes contain only few cytoplasmic filaments, well developed Golgi cisterns and normal mitochondria (Fig. 81). The filaments show diameters of 7.5–10 mμ. These cells are surrounded by numerous processes containing differing amounts of glial filaments. They form whorls and increase in number with the differentiation of the cells. The nucleus and the remain-

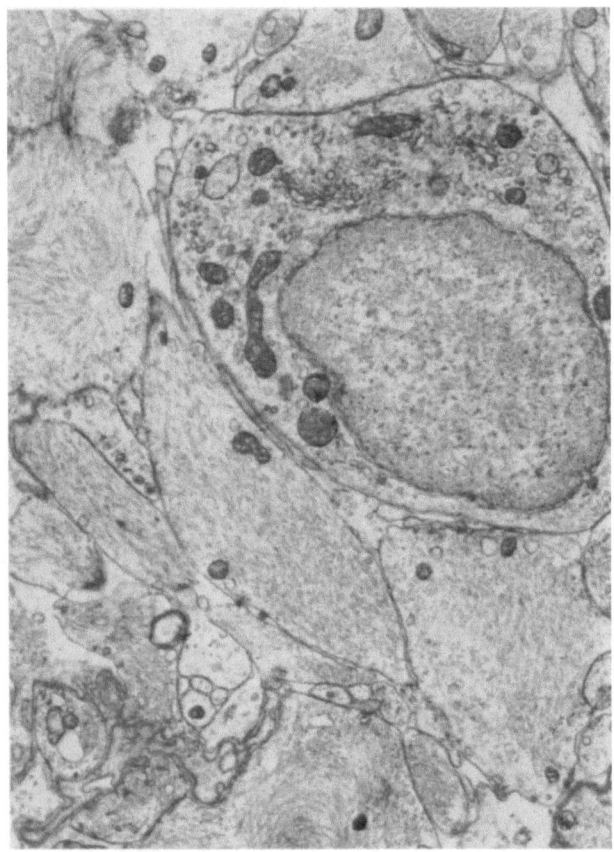

Fig. 81. Craniopharyngioma: Accumulation of glial cells in tumor center.
An undifferenciated astrocyte is surrounded by numerous processes which
are filled with glial filaments. Case 5/71, osmium, × 13,300

ing organelles are displaced towards the periphery of the cell. This
process ultimately leads to cell death. Many cell processes contain masses
of electron-dense granular material (Fig. 82). The margins of these masses
are demarcated indistinctly and are connected to the surrounding glial
filaments. The structures correspond to the Rosenthal fibers of light
microscopy and generally are judged to represent degeneration products
(Duffell *et al.*, 1963; Gullotta and Fliedner, 1972; Hossmann and Wechsler, 1965; Raimondi *et al.*, 1962; Rubinstein, 1972; Zülch and Wechsler,
1968). The glial cells of craniopharyngiomas therefore correspond to the
fibrous astrocytes of normal nervous tissue (Mugnaini and Walberg,
1964) and of astrocytomas (Poon *et al.*, 1971; Russell and Rubinstein,
1971). They can be differentiated easily from fibrillary cells of mesenchy-

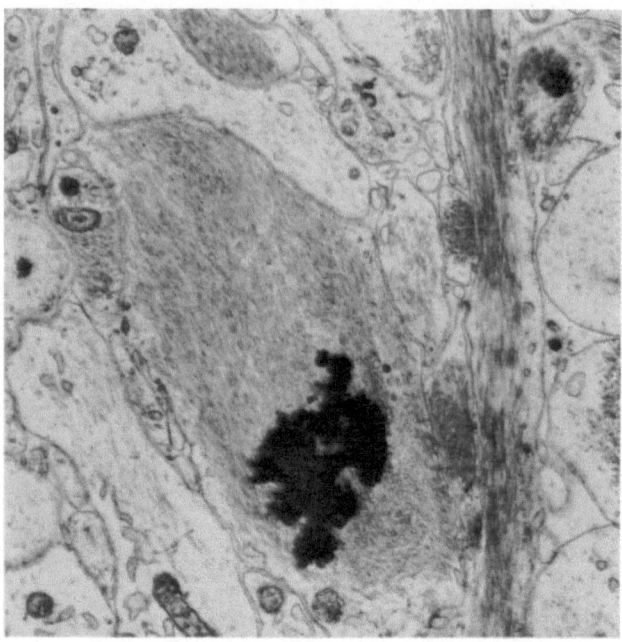

Fig. 82. Craniopharyngioma: Process of glial cell in tumor stroma demonstrating presence of Rosenthal fibers consisting of densely accumulated filaments. Case 28/72, osmium, × 13,100

mal origin. The physaliphorous cells of chordomas (Cesarini and Bonneau, 1971; Erlandson *et al.*, 1968; Friedmann *et al.*, 1962; Gessaga *et al.*, 1968; Kay and Schatzki, 1972; Pena *et al.*, 1970; Soffer *et al.*, 1970; Spjut and Luse, 1964; Wyatt *et al.*, 1971) which are located in the same region contain numerous intracytoplasmic vesicles and form microvilli on their surface. The cells of meningiomas look similar (see chapter 9) but are in immediate contact with typical collagenous fibrils. The glial cells of craniopharyngiomas are strictly separated from the collagenous tissue by an uninterrupted basal membrane (Fig. 83). Additional differences (desmosomes, pinocytotic vesicles) are obvious.

The occurrence of glia in craniopharyngiomas has been described first by Erdheim (1904). Numerous subsequent papers have confirmed the findings (del Vivo *et al.*, 1962; Ghatak *et al.*, 1971; Husten, 1923; Landolt, 1972; Russell and Rubinstein, 1971; Seemayer *et al.*, 1972). Critchley and Ironside (1926) particularly have stressed the fact that the glial tissue does not only form the tumor capsule but also can make up the bulk of the tumor. The authors report in addition that cystic cavities filled with yellow fluid can be formed by liquefaction of the neuroglia. This view has been opposed by Zülch (1956) who states that glia only

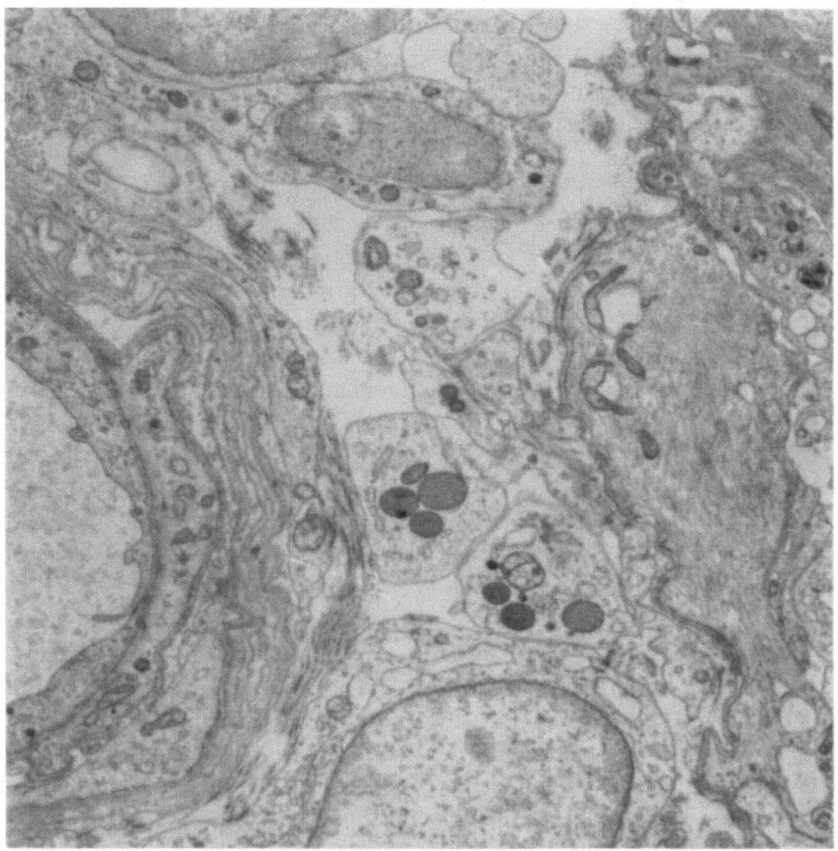

Fig. 83. Craniopharyngioma: Tumor stroma formed by capillary (left side), collagenous fibrous tissue (center), and astroglia (right side). Multiple basal membranes surround the capillary. A single, uninterrupted basal membrane separates the connective tissue and the glia. Case 11/72, osmium, × 9,500

can be present in the marginal zone of the tumor between the epithelial sprouts invading the brain. The results of tissue culture of craniopharyngiomas (Kersting, 1961; Unterharnscheidt, 1972) support this interpretation since only epithelial cells and collagenous connective tissue show active proliferation. No glia has been observed. Therefore the glia has to be judged as a product of tissue reaction (Gullotta, 1973). The negative culture results of craniopharyngioma glia might be due to technical reasons since neuroglia can be obtained from normal adult human brain tissue (Lumsden, 1971). The astroglia might be overgrown by epithelial and mesodermal cells showing a more pronounced proliferation.

The biopsies of our cases usually have been removed immediately after the surgeon's first contact with the tumor in order to get optimal quality of fixation. Using the subfrontal approach this region is usually remote from the contact zone of the tumor with the brain. The glia of our tumor biopsies therefore were situated within and not in the marginal zone of the tumor. Further evidence for this fact is presented by one of our cases (no. 29/73) containing large amounts of glia. This tumor cyst was removed easily since no adhesions existed between the neoplasm and the brain. The presence of young and fully differentiated astrocytes supports the assumption of an actively proliferating glia. Therefore we can conclude that glia are a typical but not obligatory constituent of craniopharyngiomas.

It has been assumed that craniopharyngiomas are derived from squamous epithelial rests in the region of the pars tuberalis as remnants of the embryonal Rathke's pouch (Erdheim, 1904, 1926; Russell and Rubinstein, 1971; Schurr, 1966; and others). This assumption is further substantiated by the observation of a completely intrasphenoidal cranio-pharyngioma with an intact pituitary gland; it therefore was situated in the region of the former ductus craniopharyngius (Bock, 1924). The similar structure of the enamel organ and of adamantinomas as well as the rare occurrence of tooth formation in craniopharyngiomas (see above) add further support to this view.   The experimental, intracerebral transplantation of oral epithelium produced tumors with histological characteristics of epidermoids, dermoids, and craniopharyngiomas (Van Gilder and Inukai, 1973). The incorporation of glia into an extracerebral neoplasm is only possible in congenital malformations.

Other observations suggest that craniopharyngiomas are not derived from remnants of Rathke's pouch. These remnants can be found in most normal pituitary glands and are represented by a slitlike cavity between the pars anterior and pars intermedia of the gland (Kernohan and Sayre, 1956). This cavity sometimes is lined by columnar, ciliated epithelium. This cavity remains open throughout life in the rat. Electron microscopic studies of rat tissue reveal that the anterior as well as the posterior epithelium form a continuous lining (Vanha-Perttula and Arstila, 1970). The apical surface of these cells is covered by microvilli and in some, especially posterior epithelial cells, by numerous cilia. Secretory granules are rare (Costoff, 1973), but a number of large vacuo-les can be observed.   Erdheim (1926) described a variety of epithelial types in Rathke's cyste in human autopsy material. The epithelium can be single or multilayered, cuboidal or cylindrical. The cells can show typical cilia or resemble eosinophil or basophil cells in the human adeno-hypophysis. Few intrapituitary cysts producing clinical symptoms have been reported (Duffy, 1920; Frazier and Alpers, 1934; Worster-Drought,

1934). All three cysts were lined with a single layer of columnar ciliated epithelium. The ultrastructural examination of the wall of a similar intrasellar cyst causing secondary amenorrhea in a 19 year old female in our own material showed typical adenohypophysial cells with a large number of electron dense, secretory granules and no surface specialization. The cyst was filled with cellular debris. The difference in appearance of the Rathke's pouch remnant within the pituitary gland and in the region of the pars tuberalis might therefore raise some doubts regarding the origin of the epithelial cell rests.

The squamous epithelial cell nests (Erdheim, 1904; Romeis, 1940) contain a variable number of squamous or prickle cells and are surrounded by a basal membrane. They imitate the picture of craniopharyngiomas closely but do not show signs of keratinization (Romeis, 1940). They have been observed in frequencies of 24% (Luse and Kernohan, 1955 b) up to 70% (Erdheim, 1926) in routine autopsies. Their number increases with increasing age of the patients examined. They are uncommon below the age of 20 years (Hunter, 1955) but have been found even in newborn infants (Goldberg and Eshbaugh, 1960). They have been interpreted as the results of metaplasia processes occurring in the pars tuberalis of the pituitary because of this age distribution. Squamous cell nests also have been described in the pharyngeal pituitary of normal individuals with a highly significant relationship between their incidence and the age of the patients (McPhie and Beck, 1973). Craniopharyngiomas therefore might be derived from normal pituitary cells and develop later during the life of the patient. Transitional cell forms between chromophobe cells and squamous epithelium have been described (Kernohan and Sayre, 1956). The fact that craniopharyngiomas predominate in the first two decades of life (whereas the squamous cell nests are exceedingly rare in this age group) as well as the occurrence of glia in the interior of the tumors cast some doubt on the theory that craniopharyngiomas might originate later on during life. The theory of secondary development of craniopharyngiomas from the metaplastic squamous cell nests of the pars tuberalis for this reason has to be discarded.

8. Granular Cell Tumors of the Neurohypophysis

Granular cell tumors (myoblastomas) are found in a wide variety of cutaneous, oral, and visceral sites (for review see Moscovic and Azar, 1967; Strong *et al.*, 1970). In the nervous system they have been found in the peripheral nerves (Bangle, 1953; Buldzolovich, 1968; Carstens, 1970; Fust and Custer, 1948, 1949; Garancis *et al.*, 1970), the cervical spinal leptomeninges, the cerebral hemispheres (Markesbery *et al.*, 1973), and the pituitary. Two examples of metastatic, intracerebral neoplasms believed to have been granular cell tumors have also been recorded (Meredith *et al.*, 1958; Schwidde *et al.*, 1951).—Most often granular cell tumors of the posterior lobe or of the pituitary stalk are encountered incidentally at autopsy as microscopic nodules of large, pale, granular cells. A frequency of 1.8 to 17% has been reported (Buston *et al.*, 1962; Hamperl, 1937; Harland, 1956; Kiyono, 1926; Löffler, 1929; Luse and Kernohan, 1955a; Mink *et al.*, 1955; Popovitch *et al.*, 1970; Priesel, 1922; Rap and Zarsaka, 1970; Shanklin, 1947, 1953; Simonds and Brandes, 1925; Sternberg, 1921). Occasionally they become large and produce clinical symptoms. The first such case has been described by Lüthi and Klingler (1951). Since then additional patients have been reported making up a total of 21 cases (Bara and Lantos, 1968; Burston *et al.*, 1962; Daron *et al.*, 1956; Glazer *et al.*, 1956; Harland, 1956; Jenevein, 1964; Iliescu, 1969; Korbine and Ross, 1973; Lima *et al.*, 1960; Liss and Kahn, 1958; Mink *et al.*, 1955; Poppen and Packard, 1966; Rubinstein, 1972; Satyamurti and Huntington, 1972; Sekino *et al.*, 1969; Symon *et al.*, 1971; Talerman and Dawson-Butterworth, 1966; Ulrich *et al.*, 1974).

In spite of extensive clinical and pathological investigation, including histochemical and electron microscopic studies, the histogenesis and true nature of the condition remain unknown. Theories include a non-neoplastic product of degeneration and regeneration (Ewing, 1940; Pour *et al.*, 1973; Whitten, 1968; Willis, 1960); a storage or metabolic disorder involving histiocytes (Azzopardi, 1956; Baraf and Bender, 1964; Gray and Gruenfeld, 1937; Leroux and Delarre, 1939; Shear, 1960); and a neoplasm with disturbance of metabolism of myogenic origin (Abrikossoff, 1926, 1931; Christ and Ozzello, 1971; Klemperer, 1934; Krieg, 1962; Murphy *et al.*, 1949; Murray, 1951), of neural origin (Alkek *et al.*, 1968; Ashburn and Rodger, 1952; Bangle, 1953; Carstens, 1970; Caputo *et al.*, 1972; Fisher and Wechsler, 1962; Fust and Custer, 1948, 1949; Garancis *et al.*, 1970, Sobel *et al.*, 1971, 1973b), of fibroblastic origin (Coggins, 1952; Pearse, 1950), or of mesenchymal origin (Moscovic *et al.*, 1967; Sobel *et al.*, 1973a).

We have examined material of two cases. The tissue was removed during surgery from the first and obtained at autopsy from the second. The material was fixed in unbuffered formalin in both cases before osmium fixation and plastic embedding were carried out. Both cases have been published separately.—The first patient (Ulrich et al., 1974) (no. 10/72) was a 35 year old female suffering since the age of 33 years from secondary amenorrhea and recently from a rapidly progressing organic psychosis. The neurologic examination also demonstrated a bitemporal hemianopsia. The gonadotrophin excretion was normal in spite of amenorrhea. The basal metabolic rate was decreased (–16%). The X-ray examination showed a normal sella and a suprasellar space occupying mass with compression of the third ventricle during pneumoencephalography. The CSF contained an increased protein content of 55 mg/100 ml. The solid, soft, well vascularized tumor was removed during surgery through a transventricular approach. The postoperative course was characterized by several epileptic seizures, diabetes insipidus, central hyperthermia, and electrolyte disturbances which could be controlled by appropriate fluid infusions. Three months after surgery she suffered again from an status epilepticus and died of cardiac arrest during bronchoscopy which was performed because of suspected aspiration. The autopsy showed a communicating hydrocephalus with a large opening in the floor of the third ventricle. There was no residual tumor. The pituitary was inconspicuous.

The second patient (no. 463/72) was the first case with a space occupying granular cell tumor published in the literature (Lüthi and Klingler, 1951). He survived surgery for 22 years. The detailed autopsy findings will be published elsewhere (Wegmann and Landolt, 1975).—In 1950 at the age of 34 years the patient originally was admitted to the neurosurgical clinic because of increased fatigue and slowly increasing visual disturbances. The clinical examination showed a severe visual loss on the left side with an atrophic optic papilla and bitemporal hemianopsia. There were no endocrinological symptoms. The skull X-rays showed an enlarged sella with a partially destroyed dorsum. An intrasellar tumor with suprasellar extension could be demonstrated with pneumoencephalography. The CSF protein content was reported to be normal. The solid, well vascularized tumor was removed on a transfrontal approach. After surgery the patient suffered from an pituitary insufficiency which made a full, lifelong substitution therapy with cortisone and thyroxine necessary. The postoperative diabetes insipidus of moderate severity (urine production up to 4,500 ml) disappeared spontaneously after 6 months. The patient needed psychiatric care since 1956 because of a recurrent psychosis with suicidal tendencies. In spite of this the patient was able to work as an unskilled worker performing only light work. His strength decreased somewhat in the last months of his life. He died of

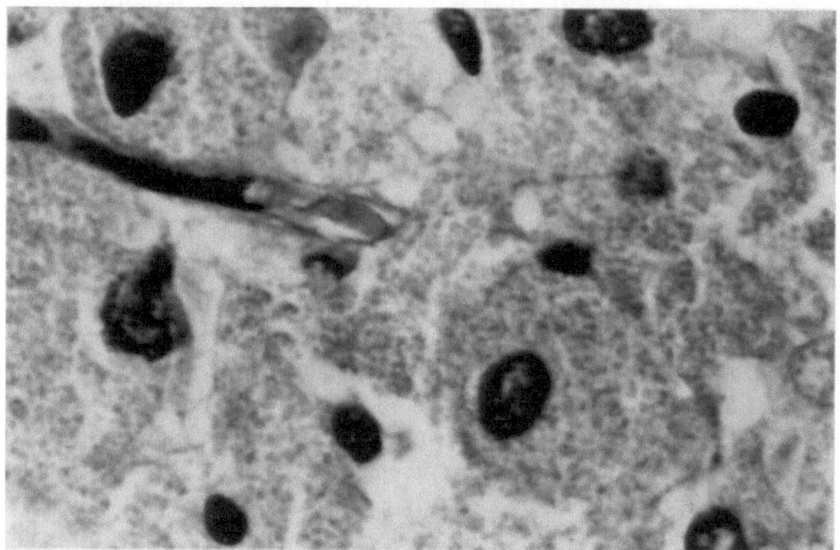

Fig. 84. Granular cell myoblastoma: Light micrograph showing densely granulated cells. The nuclei are either large and situated in the cell center or pycnotic and located at the cell periphery. Case 10/72, formalin, H & E, ×1,800

cardiac failure at the age of 56 years.—The autopsy demonstrated cardiac dilatation, chronic congestion and edema of the lungs, congestion of the spleen and kidneys, unilateral hydronephrosis, periportal fibrosis of the liver, atrophy of the thyroid, adrenals, testes, and prostate. There was a cherry sized, recurrent granular cell tumor which had not been suspected before death.

The clinical symptoms of granular cell tumors of the stalk or posterior lobe of the pituitary are those of a space occupying lesion in the region of the pituitary or the hypothalamus without signs of active hormone secretion. The most frequent symptoms concern vision (Korbine and Ross, 1973) whereas signs of adenohypophysial insufficiency are more infrequent. Preoperative diabetes insipidus (Sekino et al., 1969) and abnormal water retention (Sternberg, 1921) have been described. The skull X-rays demonstrate a normal or enlarged sella in relation to the supra- and intrasellar location of the lesion which is usually demonstrated by pneumoencephalography. Carotid angiography may show tumor stain in the pituitary region (Doron et al., 1965; Lima et al., 1960; Poppen and Packard, 1966; Symon et al., 1971). This explains the bleeding tendency of the tumors observed during surgery. The CSF protein reported in six cases is normal in two and moderately increased to

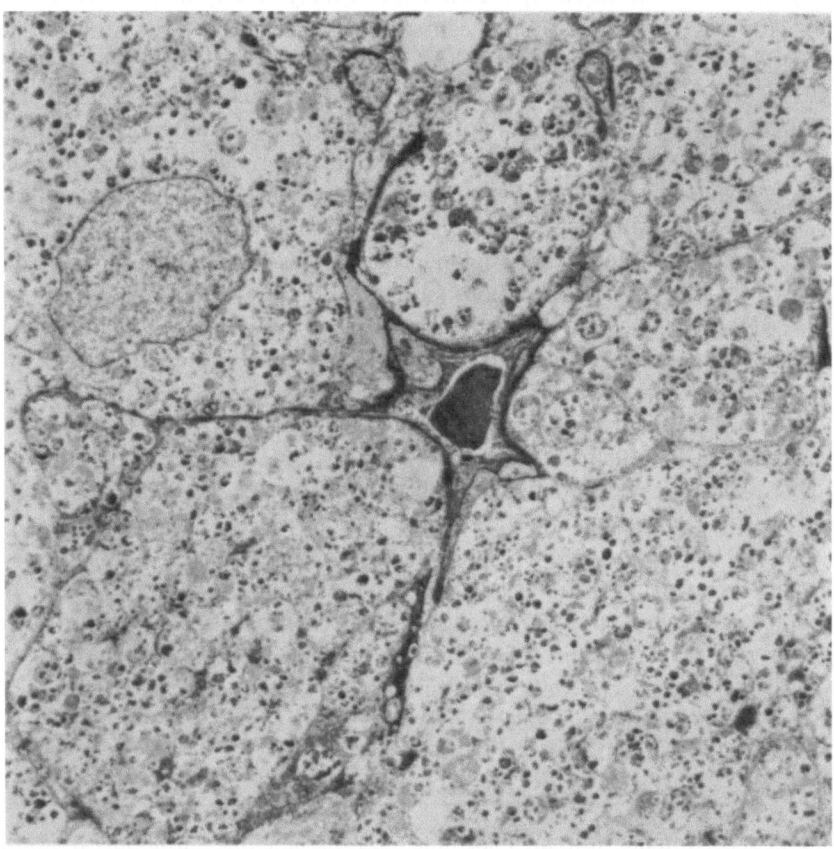

Fig. 85. Granular cell myoblastoma: Low power electron micrograph demonstrating well preserved tissue in spite of long formalin fixation. Central capillary with dense lamellae spreading in star-like fashion between the heavily granulated cells. Presence of large, round nucleus in cell center. Case 10/72, formalin-osmium, × 5,000

40–150 mg/100 ml in four.—Granular cell tumors of every localization can be treated only by excision since X-ray treatment has been found to be ineffective (Glatzer *et al.*, 1956; Jenevein, 1964; Liss and Kahn, 1958; Mink *et al.*, 1955; Satyamurti and Huntington, 1972; Strong *et al.*, 1970; Symon *et al.*, 1971).

The histological findings in all granular cell tumors whether originating in the central nervous system or of myogenous, subcutaneous, oral, or visceral origin are identical (Fig. 84). The tumors are composed of closely approximated, large, round or oval cells lacking any characteristic arrangement. Their maximum diameter is 20–45 μ. Very rarely a thin process appears to emerge from the cell body to end or pass out of the plane of section after a short course. There are two types of nuclei. The larger ones are centrally located and show a granular chromatin structure. The smaller ones have an extremely dense chromatin structure and are situated at the periphery of the cells. The most characteristic feature is the presence of an abundance of small granules in the cytoplasm. Histochemical methods demonstrate their content of proteins, lipids, and PAS-positive polysaccharides (Fisher and Wechsler, 1962; Pearse, 1950). Acid phosphatase, aminopeptidase, lipase, and unspecific esterases give strongly positive reactions (Alkek *et al.*, 1968; Whitten, 1968).

Reports concerning the ultrastructure of granular cell tumors have dealt with material originating from the urinary bladder (Christ and Ozzello, 1971), oral cavity (Fisher and Wechsler, 1962; Garancis *et al.*, 1970; Whitten, 1968), subcutaneous tissue (Caputo *et al.*, 1972; Fisher and Wechsler, 1962; Moscovic and Azar, 1967; Sobel *et al.*, 1971, 1973a), peripheral nerves (Budzilovich, 1968; Carstens, 1970; Sobel *et al.*, 1973b), brain (Markesbery *et al.*, 1973), and neurohypophysis (Popovitch *et al.*, 1970; Ulrich *et al.*, 1974). The structure of all tumors reported is basically identical. Differences reflect the various techniques used.—In spite of the fact that the surgical specimen of our first case (no. 10/72) was stored in formalin for almost five years before final processing, it still could be used to confirm the findings of the above mentioned authors. Similar observations concerning the usefulness of formalin fixated material has been collected by Hirano (1971).

Fig. 86. Granular cell myoblastoma: Desmosome-like formation between two tumor cells. Case 10/72, formalin-osmium, × 38,000

Fig. 87. Granular cell myoblastoma: Irregularly thickened cell membrane surrounding cell process containing cisterns of RER and lysosomes. Case 10/72, formalin-osmium, × 13,200

Fig. 88. Granular cell myoblastoma: Spherical granules of the first type consist of regular accumulations of microgranules and electron dense bodies of larger size. The second type of granules is represented by irregular accumulation of electron dense material between granules of first type. Case 10/72, formalin-osmium, × 15,100

Fig. 89. Granular cell myoblastoma: The third type of granule consists of irregular arrays of curvilinear material of moderate electron density. Case 10/72, formalin-osmium, × 38,400

Fig. 90. Granular cell myoblastoma: The fourth type of granule contains accumulations of myelin-like membranes and occasional dense bodies. Case 463/72, formalin-osmium, × 36,000 (electron micrograph by courtesy of Dr. W. Wegmann)

Fig. 91. Granular cell myoblastoma: Certain granules of the fourth type demonstrate arrays of parallel cristae suggesting an origin from mitochondria. Case 463/72, formalin-osmium, × 36,000 (electron micrograph by courtesy of Dr. W. Wegmann)

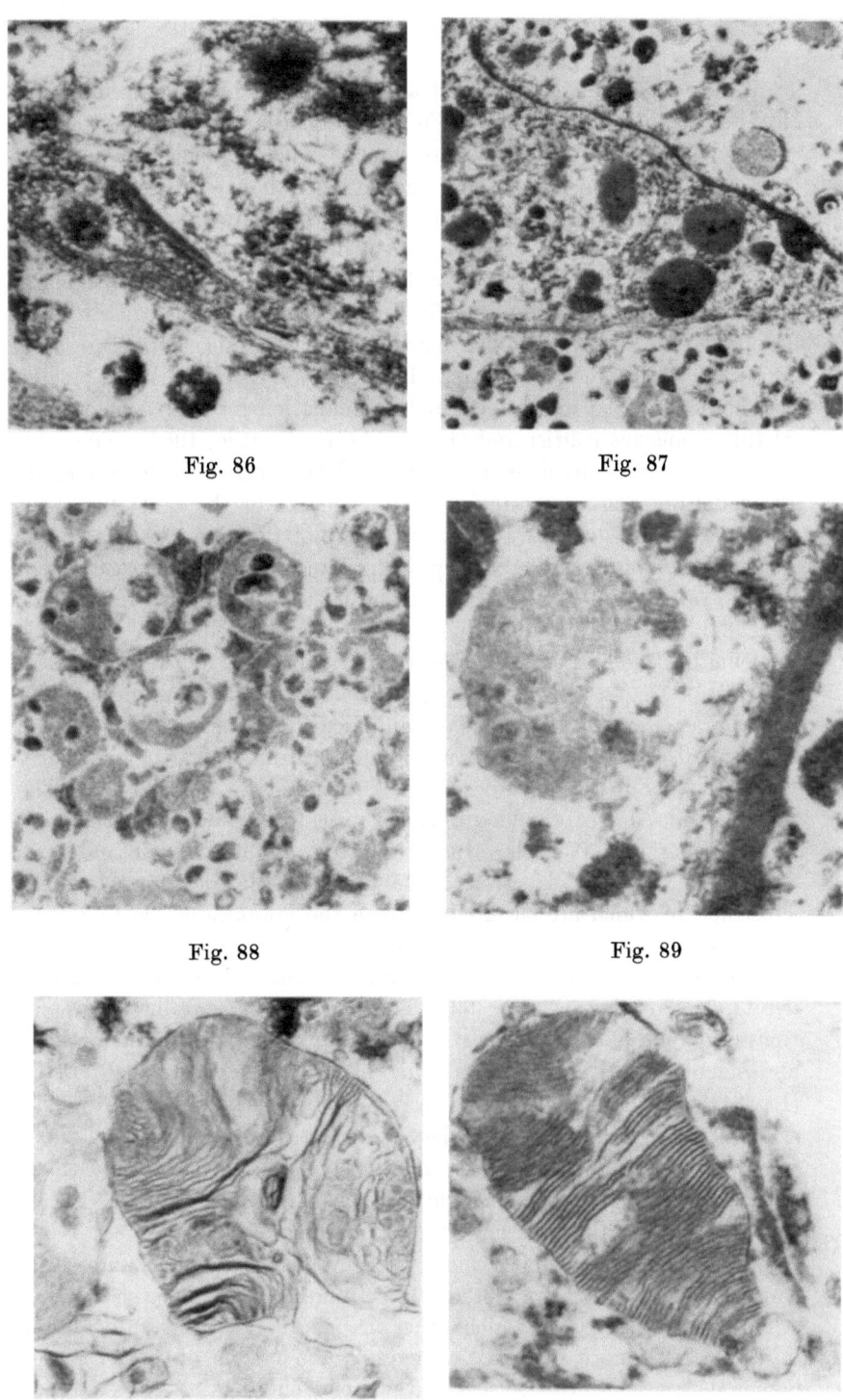

Fig. 86

Fig. 87

Fig. 88

Fig. 89

Fig. 90

Fig. 91

The round, oval or polygonal tumor cells are densely approximated leaving no intercellular space (Fig. 85). They are separated from the intercalated capillary by a dense lamella which extends between the tumor cells in a star-like manner and does not show a substructure. The large round or oval nuclei are situated in the center of the granulated cells. The cells are occasionally connected to each other by desmosome-like structures (Fig. 86). The cell membranes seem to be irregularly thickened over long distances (Fig. 87). This probably is caused by an accumulation of an intercellular substance. The presence of desmosomes in granular cell tumors of the lips, the chest wall, and the urinary bladder has been described and interpreted as indication for a myogenic origin of the neoplasms (Christ and Ozzello, 1971; Whitten, 1968). The same arguments can be used for assuming that the granular cell tumors are derived from Schwann cells or other elements of the central nervous system (Ulrich et al., 1974). The majority of the tumor cells show an accumulation of four different types of granules. The first, most frequent type shows a diameter of about 1 μ and is surrounded by a lucent halo (Fig. 88) which is probably due to a shrinkage artefact. A trace of a surrounding membrane, which is regularly present in the pictures of Christ and Ozzello (1971), can be seen occasionally. The granules contain a regular accumulation of equal sized microgranules of moderate electron density with a diameter of about 30 mμ and round, oval or irregularly shaped, electron dense bodies with a diameter of 100–320 mμ. The microgranules have been described as virus-like bodies (Caputo et al., 1972; Fisher and Wechsler, 1962; Whitten, 1968).—The second type consists of irregular, electron dense masses with occasional lamellar substructure which are situated between the granules of the first type (Fig. 88).—The third type, which has also a diameter of about 1 μ, consists of irregular arrays of circular or curvilinear formations of moderate electron density (Fig. 89). The fourth type contains accumulations of myelin-like membranes, dense bodies surrounded by membranes and microgranules (Fig. 90). Some examples show parallel cristae (Fig. 91) and therefore have been derived from mitochondria (Markesbery et al., 1973). Considering the variety of ultrastructural pictures obtained from the granules, we have to assume that they correspond to lysosomal, autophagic vacuoles digesting various cell organelles. This is further substantiated by the presence of acid phosphatase (Alkek et al., 1968; Garancis et al., 1970; Sobel et al., 1971; Whitten, 1968). Tumor cells which have not yet accumulated a large number of granules show some cell organelles (Fig. 87) which otherwise characteristically are absent from cells with more advanced changes. Some cisterns of the RER and numerous lysosomes can be seen in these elements.

The cell of origin of the granular cell tumors of the stalk and posterior

lobe of the pituitary is uncertain.—The support for a Schwann cell
origin of some of the granular cell tumors described in the literature
is based upon their occurrence in peripheral nerves (Bangle, 1953;
Buldzilovich, 1968; Carstens, 1970), the presence of axons in some
instances (Fisher and Wechsler, 1962; Garancis *et al.*, 1970, Sobel *et al.*,
1971), the existence of basement membranes about tumor cells (Caputo
et al., 1972; Fisher and Wechsler, 1962; Garancis *et al.*, 1970; Popovitch
et al., 1970; Sobel *et al.*, 1971), and the appearance of granular cells in
Schwannomas (Sobel *et al.*, 1973b). It has to be kept in mind that
myelin and myelin forming cells are extremely rare in the neurohypophysis. Romeis (1940) found only one case with myelinated nerve fibers in
the normal posterior lobe among several hundred carefully examined
pituitaries. Small nodules of granular cells are much more frequent (see
above). Liss and Kahn (1958) proposed in their comparative study that
the granular cells are derived from pituicytes, which are well known for
their tendency to accumulate iron-containing and iron-free pigment
(Romeis, 1940). Phagocytosis and lipid accumulation also has been
demonstrated in organotypic cultures of rat neural lobes (Olivieri-
Sangiacomo and Corres, 1973).—The ultrastructural examination does
not lend any support to the theory that granular cell nodules and tumors
might be derived from basophilic cells of the pars intermedia which
invaded the posterior lobe (Löffler, 1929; Shanklin, 1953) since no trace
of secretory granules can be found. The electron microscope shows also
that granular cells do not belong to the group of oncocytes as supposed
by Hamperl (1936).

The true nature of granular cell tumors of the pituitary is not known.
The above mentioned observations as well as publications of other
authors (Jenevein, 1964; Priesel, 1922; Romeis, 1940) suggest that they
originate from pituicytes and therefore cannot be classified as choristomas as Sternberg (1921) has done. In 100 serially sectioned pituitaries
Shanklin (1953) has demonstrated that nodules of granular cells (so
called "tumorettes") were not found in individuals who were younger
than 20 years. Their frequency increased from the middle age group
(18% in age 20 to 39 years) to the older age group (37.8% in age 40 to 86
years). Multiple nodules could be found in many cases with an average
of 8.5 per positive case. One case showed a total of 41 individual tumorettes. There was a definite sex relationship present with males being more
frequently affected.—These observations suggest that granular cells of
the neurohypophysis originally were a product of an age related degeneration characterized by an error of metabolism, possibly a lysosomal
defect (Garancis *et al.*, 1970). The lack of mitoses in the nodules especially
has been mentioned (Kiyono, 1926; Priesel, 1922). Cells showing this
degenerative metaplasia in the earlier phases of their ontogeny, in very

rare instances can develop autonomous growth with secondary manifestations of their metabolic disorder. Malignant growth characteristics ultimately can develop in some extremely rare cases (Al-Sarraf *et al.*, 1971; Gamboa *et al.*, 1955; Krieg, 1962; Mackenzie, 1967; Schwidde *et al.*, 1951).

The ultrastructural picture of fully developed granular cells suggests that they no longer possess the ability of mitotic division due to the lack of normal cell organelles including centrioles. Therefore we have to assume that only younger elements which occasionally can be seen give rise to the cell multiplication observed in tissue cultures of myogenic granular cell tumors (Murray, 1951).

9. Meningiomas

Meningiomas of the sellae region are characteristically situated in the area of the tuberculum sellae. Twenty-eight of 313 cases of Cushing and Eisenhardt (1938) were localized in this region. Tuberculum sellae meningiomas are about one—fifth as common as pituitary adenomas and one—half as frequent as craniopharyngiomas (Zülch, 1956). The tumors generally show a suprasellar location and grow into the sella only in the final stages.

One example from the series of the Neurosurgical Clinic in Zürich was situated entirely within the sella and did not show any connection to the tuberculum sellae (Fig. 92). The tumor had caused slowly progressive visual disturbances of four years duration. No endocrinological symptoms were noted. The exploration along the sphenoid wing demonstrated that the major part of the tumor was localized within the sella. There was a suprasellar extension which was covered by the diaphragm. The tumor compressed the optic chiasm from below.

The electron micrographs of this intrasellar tumor show blastomatous elements, connective-vascular tissue, and mast cells. This tumor belongs to the group of endotheliomatous meningiomas (Zülch 1956) and consists of a compact accumulation of cell bodies with numerous processes (Fig. 93). The ultrastructure corresponds to that of other meningiomas (Castaigne et al., 1966; Cervos-Navarro, 1967; Cervos-Navarro and Vazquez, 1966, 1969; Escourolle and Poirier, 1971; Keepes, 1961; Long, 1973; Luse, 1960; Nyström, 1965, 1973; Poon et al., 1971; Raimondi et al., 1962; Robertson, 1964; Rubinstein, 1972; Russell and Rubinstein, 1971). The nuclei are generally round or slightly elongated. They are regular in shape and well delineated. Some nuclei are grooved to varying depths. Deep fissures give origin to the "eosinophilic nuclear inclusions" of light microscopy if sectioned appropriately (Robertson, 1964). The chromatin structure is finely granular. Nucleoli can be observed. The cytoplasm is characterized by irregular protrusions. The main part of the cytoplasm is occupied by innumerable microfibrils measuring about 5 mμ in diameter (Fig. 94). The fibrils can be irregularly arranged or run in whorls and parallel arrays. They can be condensed and form structures like Rosenthal fibers (compare page 115) (Raimondi et al., 1962). Mitochondria, Golgi structures, and the RER are generally accumulated in regions close to the nucleus. Lipid inclusions and myelin bodies can occasionally be observed. Pinocytotic vesicles are abundant and characteristic for meningiomas. Intracytoplasmic cilia occasionally can be seen (Cervos-Navarro, 1967; Cervos-Navarro and Vazquez, 1966). Their presence does not necessarily mean that the cells originate from epithelial cells since they have been described in mesenchymal elements too

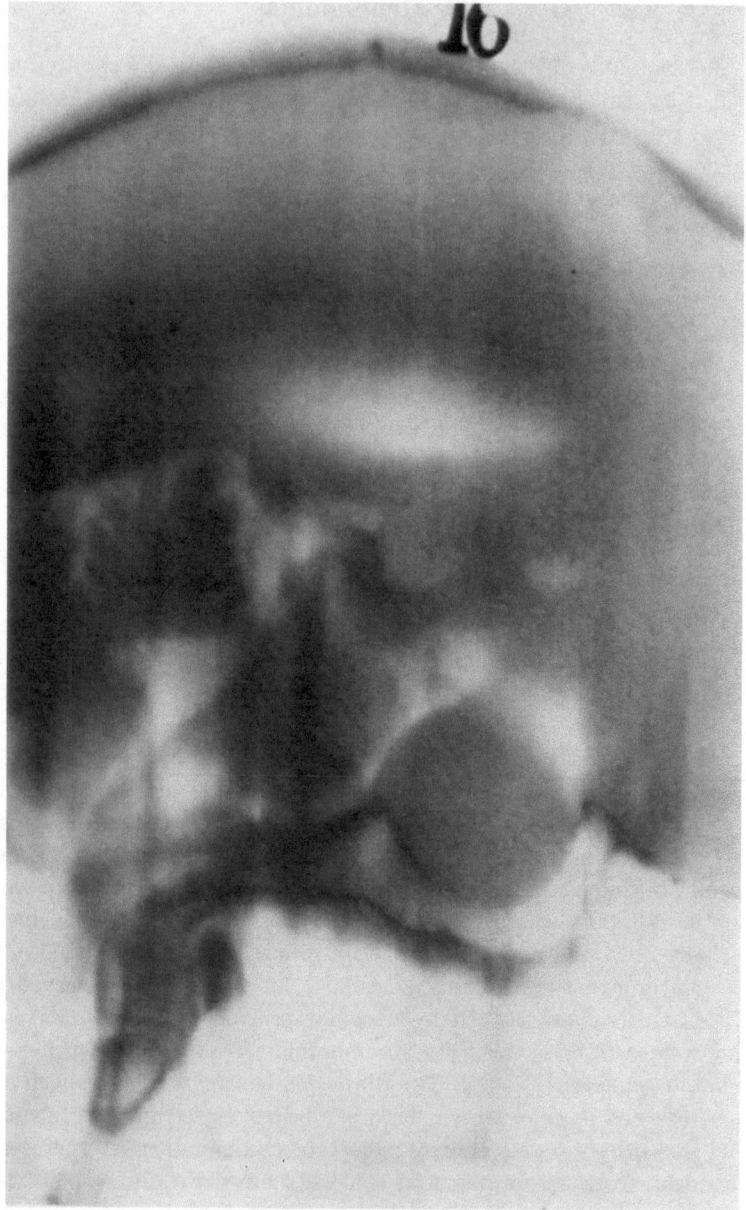

Fig. 92. Intrasellar meningioma: Sagittal tomogram of air study demonstrating entirely intrasellar location of tumor without connections to tuberculum
sellae (radiograph by courtesy of Dr. H. Etter). Case 51/72

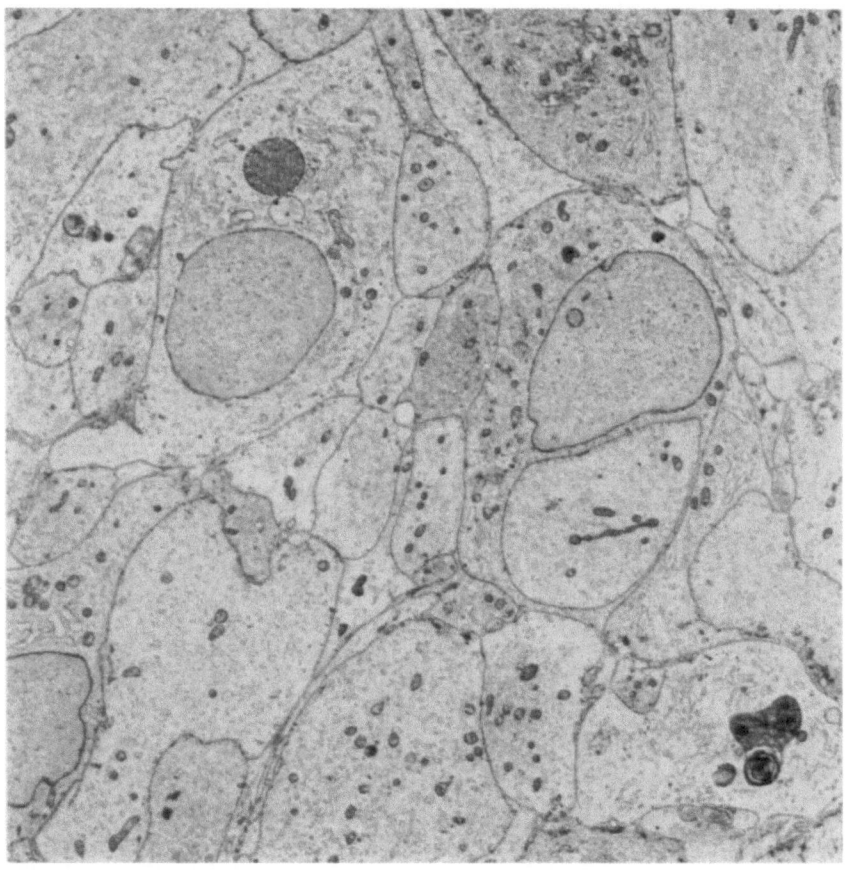

Fig. 93. Intrasellar meningioma: Tumor consisting of dense accumulation of polygonal cell bodies with large homogenous nuclei and numerous interwoven cell processes with occasional lipid and myelin bodies. Case 51/72, osmium, × 4,300

(Sorokin, 1962). Numerous desmosomes and occluding zones which connect the tumor cells to each other complete the picture (Fig. 94). They are particularly abundant in cells rich in cytofilaments which are often connected with them.

Light microscopy differentiates at least three types of meningiomas: endotheliomateus, fibrous, angiomatous type (Zülch 1956). The electron microscope demonstrates that all three are composed of the same cell type (Cervos-Navarro and Vazquez, 1964; Escourolle and Poirier, 1971; Nyström, 1965). The histological difference is caused only by different cell texture and differing amounts of collagen fibres and capillaries.

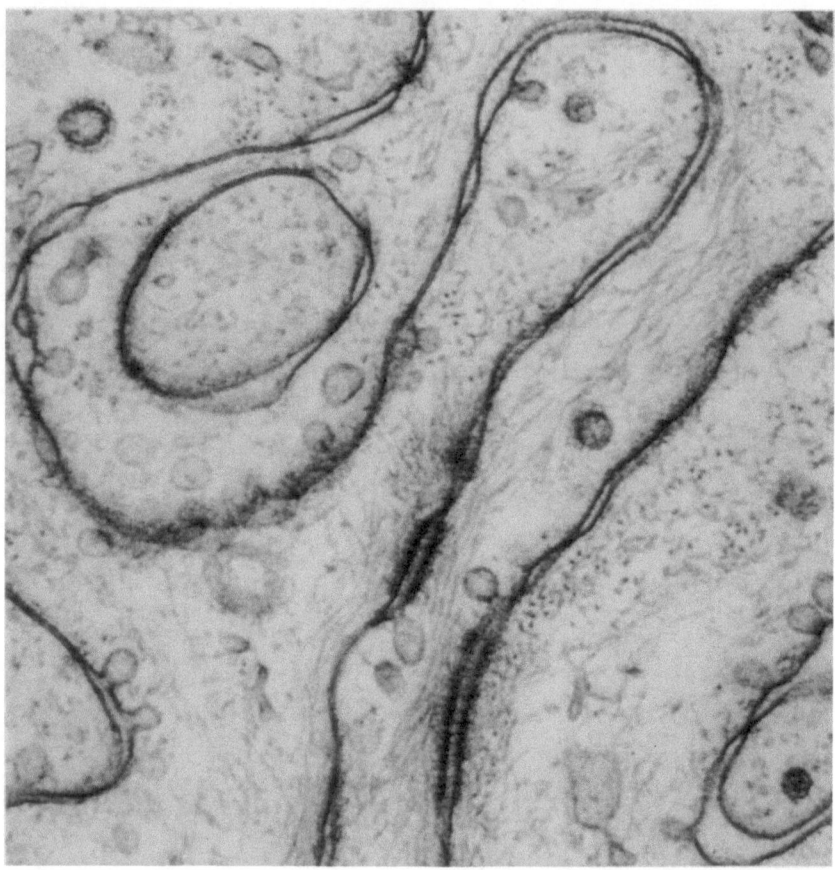

Fig. 94. Intrasellar meningioma: The cell processes contain loosely arranged fibrils originating from desmosomes. Some pinocytotic vesicles can be observed. Case 51/72, osmium, × 61,000

All cellular elements of meningiomas resemble closely the cell clusters capping the arachnoid villi and the cell inclusions which are found in increasing numbers as age advances, between the fibrous strands of the dura mater (Cushing and Eisenhardt, 1938; Schmidt, 1902). The affinity of meningiomas for the dural sinuses has long been recognized. Meningiomas may, however, arise from arachnoid cells anywhere along the arachnoid membrane. The arachnoid cells along the surface of the diaphragm of the sella invade the opening of the dura in the region of the pituitary stalk and have close connections to the connective tissue of the pituitary surface. The arachnoid forms a diverticulum which is in close contact with the pituitary body (Romeis, 1940). The intrasellar meningioma described therefore seems to originate from this arachnoid pocket. This is further substantiated by the fact that the bony floor of the sella is not covered by dura but rather by a periosteum showing an entirely different histological structure (Romeis, 1940).

The ultrastructure examination of normal arachnoid of man and different mammals (Andres, 1967 a, b; Jayatilaka, 1965; Pease and Schulz, 1958; Ramsey, 1965; Waggener and Beggs, 1967) shows overlapping cells with connective tissue trabecules. The plasmalemmas are separated sporadically by extracellular lacunae containing collagen fibrils. The cells are not as flat as those of the dura. In addition to numerous mitochondria, a variety of other cell organelles is well represented. The Golgi complex is prominent and frequently occupies the perinuclear zone. Clusters of endoplasmic reticulum are arranged in short profiles. Ribosomal rosettes and microfibrils are dispersed within the cytoplasmic matrix. Lysosomes and lipid bodies are encountered. The plasmalemma is invaginated at intervals to form pinocytotic and coated vesicles. The nuclei are elongated and show numerous indentations. The plasma membranes generally show a uniform, electron lucent gap of approximately 20 mµ. However, this simple arrangement is frequently interrupted by focal junctional complexes which include desmosomes (macula adhaerens) and external compound membranes (zonula occludens) (Brightman and Palay, 1963; Farquhar and Palade, 1963). Meningiomas show the same main features as do normal arachnoid cells: indented nuclei, intracellular fibrils, pinocytotic vesicles and junctional complexes. This demonstrates the origin of meningiomas from arachnoid cells on an ultrastructural level.

10. Summary

The original three cell type classification (eosinophilic, basophilic, chromophobe) of the pituitary has been invalidated by modern staining techniques and more recently by immunohistologic procedures. The resultant observations led to the establishment of the "one cell, one hormone" theory indicating that each pituitary hormone (somatotrophic, thyrotrophic, adrenocorticotrophic, melanotrophic, lactogenic) with the exeption of the two gonadotrophic hormones is produced by a particular cell type characterized by distinct staining properties. The two gonadotrophic hormones (follicle stimulating and luteinizing hormone) are probably produced by the same cell.—The ultrastructural examination of the *normal human anterior pituitary* led to the same conclusion. Differences in cell size and shape, number, distribution and morphology of granules in the cytoplasm and amount of rough-surfaced endoplasmic reticulum are all used to distinguish the individual cell types. The exact correlation of each hormone with its production site has been established only in experimental animals and no unanimity has been reached for all cell types in man. Several publications agree only in the description of three cells (somatotrophic, prolactin producing, thyrotrophic).—In addition to the six granulated hypophysial cells involved in hormone production there are nongranulated cells, which are involved in the delineation of the colloid containing follicles. These follicular cells have star-like processes which extend between the secretory cells. There is no evidence to suggest hormone production in the follicular cells. They seem to represent the only true chromophobe cell since the staining characteristics observed with modern staining methods is dependent upon the stored hormone granules.

The secretory process is similar in all pituitary parenchymal cells. The different hormones are synthesized in the cisterns of the rough-surfaced endoplasmic reticulum, and transported to the Golgi cisterns where they are condensed and packed into vesicles forming dense cored granules. The granules grow by fusion and are transformed into characteristic ripe granules which assemble beneath the cell membrane before extrusion takes place. Sudden suppression of stimulated hormone secretion results in destruction of the accumulated secretory granules in lysosomes.

The *pars intermedia of the normal pituitary* has been examined only in experimental animals. Two granulated cell types, related to ACTH and MSH production respectively, are noted. The third cell type is agranular and occurs either as a follicular cell or as a marginal cell which forms a continuous lining of the pituitary cleft if present. Numerous nerve endings can be observed forming contacts with the granulated cells.

The *normal neurohypophysis* contains pituicytes with large nuclei, relatively scarce perinuclear cytoplasm, and numerous slender processes which intermingle with nerve fibers. The number of elementary granules and empty vesicles in these fibers can be altered by salt loading, dehydration and acute bleeding.

Pituitary adenomas form the largest number of human sellar tumors and can be easily divided into two groups: The first presents clinical signs of endocrinological hyperactivity, the second exhibits signs of a space occupying lesion associated with varying degrees of hypopituitarism. The first group (hypersecretion) is further divided into subgroups characterized by the particular endocrinological syndromes of hypersomatotropism, hyperprolactinism, hyperadrenocorticism and hyperthyrotropism.

Acromegaly is produced by densely granulated ("eosinophilic") or sparsely granulated ("chromophobe") adenomas. Intermediary forms exist. The sparsely granulated specimens contain considerably smaller granules than the more heavily granulated ones. Granule size distribution curves show that, contrary to the normal gland, there is no "typical HGH granule" in the adenomas. The abnormal tissue produces abnormal granules. Other cytological features (fibril accumulation, follicle formation) can be used for the differentiation of typical hormone secreting adenomas. Almost one third of the adenomas associated with acromegaly show virus-like tubular structures in the perinuclear cisterns of the endothelial cells.

Comparison of the preoperative serum HGH level with granule size shows that the rapidity of granule formation varies considerably. Several different ultrastructural parameters can be combined in order to obtain a morphological "activity index" which can be related to the preoperative serum HGH level. An agreement of the relative values can be observed in the majority of cases. Some differences can be explained by the observation that certain adenomas produce HGH and LTH simultaneously. Similar observations can be made in cases of *Forbes-Albright syndrome* which is caused by a LTH producing adenoma.

Two types of adenomas have been described with *Cushing's and Nelson's syndrome*. One type demonstrates Crooke's hyalin changes, the other does not. There is no relationship between the two clinical and ultrastructural entities nor with that of ACTH- or MSH-production. The hormone granules of adenomas without Crooke's cells show a tendency to disrupt during direct osmium fixation. This fact, as well as the formation of Cooke's fibrils, has been related to MSH-production by various authors. Our own observation suggest that this assumption is probably not valid in neoplastic tissue. We have examined a pituitary adenoma in a case of longstaining *Addison's disease* with increased ACTH secretion, and found it to consist mainly of Crooke's cells.

Thyrotrophic adenomas of the pituitary are observed in cases of long-standing myxedema and in patients with Grave's disease which disappears after removal of the adenoma. This suggests that the hyperthyroidism is secondary to the increased TSH secretion whereas tumors with hypothyroidism are probably due to increased hypothalamic stimulation. Results of the ultrastructural examination have only been reported in a single case with Grave's disease.

The majority of pituitary adenomas do not show clinical evidence of hormone secretion. They are usually designated as "chromophobe adenomas". It is suggested for a number of reasons that this misleading term be replaced by "endocrine inactive adenomas". Ultrastructural examination shows this to be a rather mixed and varied group of tumors.

Oncocytomas consist of finely granulated eosinophilic cells with a swollen appearance. This fine granulation is caused by a dense accumulation of abnormal mitochondria. Secretory granules are extremely rare. Oncocytes of pituitary adenomas as well as oncocytes from other organs and tumors seem to suffer from a defective oxidative metabolism and are therefore probably unable to synthesize their normal secretory. They are slow growing tumors.

Most cases of *endocrine inactive adenomas* show ultrastructural features of ongoing secretory processes. Almost every tumor contains granulated cells. Prolactin may be secreted by a number of adenomas in spite of the absence of galactorrhea. This is demonstrated by high serum LTH levels in cases without Forbes-Albright syndrome. Clinical evidence for "silent" LTH production can also be gained from the observation of a Peillon-Racadot syndrome. These female patients with secondary amenorrhea, react to treatment with estrogens with headaches and visual symptoms caused by the stimulated growth of a previously undetected pituitary adenoma.—Other adenomas show ultrastructural signs of STH production in spite of the absence of clinical features of acromegaly. The production rate of the hormone may be so low that it is still within normal limits and therefore does not cause clinical evidence of the disease. The frequently observed process of crinophagy may further influence the amount of hormones ultimately secreted. Some rare adenomas show, in addition to granulated cells, large numbers of follicular cells which are probably not capable of producing hormones.

It is therefore suggested that basically all pituitary adenomas belong to one of the subgroups mentioned which show endocrine activity. The amount of hormone secreted may vary from very high levels to within normal limits. Some morphological signs of the varying activity can be seen in the electron micrographs of the various adenomas. It has been shown that certain cell organelles contribute to hormone synthesis (mitochondria, rough-surfaced endoplasmic reticulum, Golgi cisterns) whereas others are engaged in hormone destruction (lysosomes) or hormone retention (cell membrane). The amount of hormone ultimately reaching the blood stream may be only a small fraction of that originally synthesized. Variations in the amount synthesised may be due not only to the differing development of the rough-surfaced endoplasmic reticulum but also to degenerative changes in mitochondria leading to the formation of oncocytes.

Malignant pituitary adenomas or carcinomas are extremely rare. The most frequent sign of aggressive growth is that of local invasion. Tumors with subarachnoidal or hematogenous metastases are even rarer but often show (17 of 25 cases collected from the literature) signs of endocrine hyperactivity. Ultrastructural examination of five tumors with invasive growth did not demonstrate any obvious difference when compared to noninvasive adenomas.

The ultrastructural examination of *craniopharyngiomas* demonstrates that the tumor consists of epithelial cells, collagenous tissue, blood vessels, and fibrillary glia which is a typical but not obligatory constituent, all of which are strictly separated from each other by continuous basement membranes. Epithelium, connective tissue and glia show characteristic processes of differentiation and degeneration leading to the formation of parakeratotic masses, heterotopic calcification, cysts, pseudocysts, and Rosenthal fibers.

Granular cell tumors of the neurohypophysis are extremely rare. Ultrastructural findings have previously been reported in only two cases. The rather large cells contain several types of composite cytoplasmic granules. Some of these resemble altered mitochondria, others lysosomes. Granular cell tumors of other tissue origin (urinary bladder, oral cavity, subcutaneous tissue, peripheral nerve, brain) show a basically similar structure. The granular cells in tumors of the neurohypophysis are probably derived from pituicytes.

Meningiomas of the sella region usually originate from the tuberculum sellae. The ultrastructural findings in a meningioma which was situated entirely within the sella is described. This peculiar location suggests that it originated from the arachnoidal cells forming a diverticulum in the opening of the diaphragm.

References

Abrams, H. L., Spiro, R., Goldstein, N. (1950), Metastases in carcinoma. Analysis of 100 autopsied cases. Cancer *3*, 74—85.

Abrikossoff, A. (1926), Über Myome ausgehend von der quergestreiften willkürlichen Muskulatur. Virchow's Arch. *260*, 215—233.

— (1931), Weitere Untersuchungen über Myoblastenmyome. Virchow's Arch. *280*, 723—740.

Albeaux-Fernet, M., Guiot, J., Braun, S., Cauvin, R., Romani, J. D. (1955), Exophthalmie oedémateuse maligne traitée par hypophysectomie. Présence d'une hyperplasie cyanophile à cellules delta sur les coupes. Bull. Mém. Soc. Hôp. Paris *71*, 220—229.

Alkek, D. S., Johnson, W. C., Graham, J. H. (1968), Granular cell myoblastoma. A histological and enzymatic study. Arch. Derm. (Chicago) *98*, 543—547.

Allanson, M., Forster, C. L., Cameron, E. (1969), Mitotic activity in the adenohypophysis of pregnant and lactating rabbits. J. Reprod. Fertil. *19*, 121—131.

Al-Sarraf, M., Loud, A. V., Vaitkevicius, V. K. (1971), Malignant granular cell tumor. Histochemical and electron microscopic study. Arch. Path. (Chicago) *91*, 550—558.

Andersen, H., Bülow, F. A. von, Møllgård, K. (1970), The histochemical and ultrastructural basis of the cellular function of the human foetal adenohypophysis. Progr. Histochem. Cytochem. *1*, 153—184.

Anderson, C. H., Kim, B., Minkowitz, S. (1969), Calcifying epithelial odontogenic tumor of Pindborg. An electron microscopic study. Cancer *24*, 585—596.

Anderson, W. A. D. (1953), Pathology. 2nd ed. London: H. Kimpton.

Andres, K. H. (1967 a), Über die Feinstruktur der Arachnoidea und Dura mater von Mammalia. Z. Zellforsch. *79*, 272—295.

— (1967 b), Zur Feinstruktur der Arachnoidalzotten bei Mammalia. Z. Zellforsch. *82*, 92—109.

Ashburn, L. L., Rodger, R. C. (1952), Myoblastomas, neural origin. Report of six cases, one with multiple tumors. Amer. J. Clin. Path. *22*, 440—448.

Askanazy, M. (1898), Pathologisch-anatomische Beiträge zur Kenntnis des Morbus Basedowi, insbesondere über die dabei auftretende Muskelerkrankung. Dtsch. Arch. klin. Med. *61*, 118—186.

Azzopardi, J. G. (1956), Histogenesis of the granular-cell "myoblastoma". J. Path. Bact. *71*, 85—93.

Backlund, E.-O. (1973), Studies on craniopharyngiomas: III. Stereotaxic treatment with intracystic Yttrium-90. Acta Chir. Scand. *139*, 237—247.

Bahn, R. C., Ross, G. T., MacCarty, C. S. (1960), Melanocyte stimulating hormone and ACTH activities of pituitary tumors in patients with Cushing's syndrome. Proc. Mayo Clin. *35*, 623—629.

Bailey, O. T., Cutler, E. C. (1940), Malignant adenomas of the chromophobe cells of the pituitary body. Arch. Path. (Chicago) *29*, 368—399.

Bailey, P. (1932), Tumors of the hypophysis cerebri. In: W. Penfield (ed.): Cytology and cellular pathology of the nervous system, p. 905—951. New York: Hoeber.

— Buchanan, D. N., Bucy, P. C. (1939), Intracranial tumors in infancy and childhood. Chicago: University of Chicago Press.

Bailey, P., Cushing, H. (1928), Studies in acromegaly. VII. The microscopical structure of the adenomas in acromegalic dyspituitarism (fugitive acromegaly). Amer. J. Path. *4*, 545—563.

Bakay, L. (1950), The results of 300 pituitary adenoma operations. J. Neurosurg. *7*, 240—255.

Baker, B. L., Yu, Y.-Y. (1971), The thyrotropic cell of the rat hypophysis as studied with peroxidase-labeled antibody. Amer. J. Anat. *131*, 55—72.

Balogh, K., Jr., Cohen, R. B. (1961), Oxydative enzymes in epithelial cells of normal and pathological human parathyroid glands: A histochemical study. Lab. Invest. *10*, 354—360.

— Roth, S. I. (1965), Histochemical and electron microscopic studies of eosinophilic granular cells (oncocytes) in tumors of the parotid gland. Lab. Invest. *14*, 310—320.

Bancroft, F. C., Tashjian, A. H., Jr. (1970), Control of the production of two protein hormones by rat pituitary cells in culture. In Vitro *6*, 180—189.

Bangle, R. (1953), An early granular-cell myoblastoma confined within a small peripheral myelinated nerve. Cancer *6*, 790—793.

Bara, D., Lantos, P. (1968), Two rare forms of tumour in the hypothalamo-hypophysial system. Infundibular choristoma and glioblastoma infiltrating the pituitary. Acta morph. Acad. Sci. Hung. *16*, 243—250.

Baraf, C. S., Bender, B. (1964), Multiple cutaneous granular cell myoblastoma. Arch. Derm. (Chicago) *89*, 243—246.

Bargmann, W., Lindner, E., Andres, K. H. (1967), Über Synapsen an endokrinen Epithelzellen und die Definition sekretorischer Neurone. Untersuchungen am Zwischenlappen der Katzenhypophyse. Z. Zellforsch. *77*, 282—298.

Barnes, B. G. (1961), Ciliated secretory cells in the pars distalis of the mouse hypophysis. J. Ultrastruct. Res. *5*, 453—467.

— (1962), Electron microscope studies on the secretory cytology of the mouse anterior pituitary. Endocrinology *71*, 618—628.

— (1963), The fine structure of the mouse adenohypophysis in various physiological states. In: J. Benoit, C. Da Lage (eds.): Cytologie de l'adénohypophyse. Editions du Centre National de la Recherche Scientifique, Paris.

Beck, H. (1883), Über ein Teratom der Hypophysis cerebri. Heilkunde *4*, 393—409.

Benoit, J., Da Lage, C. (eds.) (1963), Cytologie de l'adénophyophyse. Editions du Centre National de la Recherche Scientifique, Paris.

Bergland, R. M., Torack, R. M. (1969a), An ultrastructural study of follicular cells in the human anterior pituitary. Amer. J. Path. *57*, 273—297.

— — (1969b), Microtubules and neurofilaments in axons of the human pituitary stalk. Exp. Cell Res. *54*, 132—134.

— — (1969c), An electron microscopic study of the human infundibulum. Z. Zellforsch. *99*, 1—12.

Blackwood, W., McMenemey, W. H., Meyer, A., Norman, R. M., Russell, D. S. (1963), Greenfield's Neuropathology, 2nd ed., p. 456—457. London: E. Arnolds.

Bock, E. (1924), Beitrag zur Pathologie der Hypophyse. Virochow's Arch. *252*, 98—112.

Braun, W., Tzonos, T. (1965), Über ein ungewöhnlich rasch wachsendes Hypophysencarcinom mit intracerebralen Metastasen. Acta Neurochir. (Wien) *12*, 615—624.

Bricaire, H., Luton, J. P., Turpin, G. (1973), Tumeurs de l'hypophyse et syndromes de Cushing. Nouv. Presse Méd. *2*, 499—502.

Brightman, M. W., Palay, S. L. (1963), The fine structure of ependyma of the rat brain. J. Cell Biol. *19*, 415—439.

Brion, S., Fanjoux, J. (1958), Histologie. In: G. Guiot (ed.): Adénomes Hypophysaires, p. 142—156. Paris: Masson.

Brody, I. (1960), The ultrastructure of tonofibrilis in the keratinization process of normal human epidermis. J. Ultrastruct. Res. *4*, 264—297.

— (1962a), The ultrastructure of the epidermis in psoriasis vulgaris as revealed by electron microscopy. 1. The dermo-epidermal junction and the stratum basale in parakeratosis without keratohyalin. J. Ultrastruct. Res. *6*, 304—323.

— (1962b), The ultrastructure of the epidermis in psoriasis vulgaris as revealed by electron microscopy. 4. Stratum corneum in parakeratosis without keratohyalin. J. Ultrastruct. Res. *6*, 354—367.

Brown, W. L. (1925), Discussion on the uses and abuses of endocrine therapy. Brit. Med. J. *2*, 1051—1056.

Brucher, J. M., Soffer, D., Wechsler, W. (1970), Feinstruktur eines polymorphen Hypophysenadenoms. Path. Europ. *5*, 442—453.

Budzilovich, G. N. (1968), Cranular cell "myoblastoma" of vagus nerve. Acta Neuropath. (Berlin) *10*, 162—165.

Burston, J., John, R., Spencer, H. (1962), "Myoblastoma" of the neurohypophysis. J. Path. Bact. *83*, 455—461.

Cagnetto, G. (1904), Zur Frage der anatomischen Beziehung zwischen Akromegalie und Hypophysistumor. Virchow's Arch. *176*, 115—168.

Cairns, H., Russell, D. S. (1931), Intracranial and spinal metastases in gliomas of the brain. Brain *54*, 376—420.

Cameron, G. R. (1952), Pathology of the cell. Edinburgh: Oliver and Boyd.

Cancilla, P., Morecki, R., Hurwitt, E. S. (1964), Fine structure of a recurrent chordoma. Arch. Neurol. (Chicago) *11*, 289—295.

Caputo, R., Bellone, A. G., Tagliavini, R. (1972), Ultrastructure of the granular cell myoblastoma. So-called Abrikossoff's tumor. Arch. Derm. Forsch. *242*, 127—136.

Cardell, R. R. (1963), The cytophysiology of the anterior pituitary gland. Henry Ford Hosp. Med. Bull. *11*, 409—430.

— Knighton, R. S. (1966), The cytology of a human pituitary tumor: an electron microscopic study. Trans. Amer. Microsc. Soc. *85*, 58—78.

Carstens, P. H. B. (1970), Ultrastructure of granular cell myoblastoma. Acta Path. Microbiol. Scand. *78*, 685—694.

Castaigne, P., Escourolle, R., Poirier, J. (1966), L'ultrastructure des méningiomes. Etude de 4 cas en microscopie électronique. Rev. Neurol. (Paris) *114*, 249—261.

Caughey, J. E., Lester, M. J. (1961), Hyothyroidism and pituitary tumours. New Zeal. Med. J. *60*, 486—489.

Cervos-Navarro, J. (1967), Zur Feinstructur endotheliomatöser Meningeome des Menschen. Acta Neuropath. (Berl.) *8*, 141—148.

— Vazquez, J. (1966), Elektronenmikroskopische Untersuchungen über das Vorkommen von Cilien in Meningeomen. Virchow's Arch. *341*, 280—290.

Cervos-Navarro, J., Vazquez, J. (1969), An electron microscopic study of meningiomas. Acta Neuropath. (Berl.) *13*, 301—323.

Cesarini, J.-P., Bonneau, H. (1971), A propos de l'étude ultrastructurale d'un chordome sacré. Arch. Anat. Path. (Paris) *19*, 95—102.

Chaudhry, A. P., Hanks, C. T., Leifer, C., Garguglio, E. A. (1972), Calcifying epithelial odontogenic tumor. Cancer *30*, 519—529.

Christ, M. L., Ozzello, L. (1971), Myogenous origin of a granular cell tumor of the urinary bladder. Amer. J. Clin. Path. *56*, 736—749.

Coggins, R. P. (1952), Granular-cell myoblastoma of common bile duct. Report of a case with autopsy findings. Arch. Path. (Chicago) *54*, 398—402.

Cohen, H., Dible, J. H. (1936), Pituitary basophilism associated with a basophil carcinoma of the anterior lobe of the pituitary gland. Brain 395—407.

Committee on medical rating of physical impairment (1958), Guides to the evaluation of permanent impairment: The visual system. J. A. M. A. *168*, 475—488.

Connolly, C., Connell, A. M. S. (1958), The effects of section of the pituitary stalk in malignant disease. Brit. J. Surg. *46*, 118—121.

Contopoulos, A. N., Simpson, M. E., Koneff, A. A. (1958), Pituitary function in the thyroidectomized rat. Endocrinology *63*, 642—653.

Cooper, J. R. (1967), Tumor tissue growth. The growth of tumor tissues from the central nervous system in tissue culture. J. Kansas Med. Soc. *68*, 340—343.

Costoff, A. (1973), Ultrastructure of rat adenohypophysis.—Correlation with function. New York: Academic Press.

Cottier, H. (1966), Histopathologie der Wirkung ionisierender Strahlen auf höhere Organismen. In: L. Diethelm, O. Olsson, F. Strnad, H. Vieten und A. Zuppinger: Handbuch der medizinischen Radiologie, Vol. II/2. Berlin-Heidelberg-New York: Springer.

Cowie, A. T. (1966), Anterior pituitary function in lactation. In: G. W. Harris, B. T. Donovan (eds.): The pituitary gland. Vol. 2. London: Butterworths.

Critchley, M., Ironside, R. N. (1926), The pituitary adamantinomata. Brain *49*, 357—481.

Crompton, M. R., Layton, D. D. (1961), Delayed radionecrosis of the brain following therapeutic x-radiation of the pituitary. Brain *84*, 85—101.

Crooke, A. C. (1935), A change in the basophil cells of the pituitary gland common to conditions which exhibit the syndrome attributed to basophil adenoma. J. Path. Bact. *41*, 339—349.

Curé, M., Trouillas, J., Lhéritier, M., Girod, C., Rollet, J. (1972), Inclusions tubulaires dans une tumeur hypophysaire. Nouv. Presse Méd. *1*, 2309—2311.

Cushing, H. (1912), The pituitary body and its disorders. (Clinical states produced by disorders of the hypophysis cerebri.) Philadelphia: J. B. Lippincott Company.

— (1932a), The basophil adenomas of the pituitary body and their clinical manifestations (pituitary basophilism). In: Papers relating to the pituitary body, hypothalamus and parasympathetic nervous system. Springfield: Ch. C Thomas.

Cushing, H. (1932b), Intracranial tumors. Notes upon a series of two thousand verified cases with surgical mortality percentages pertaining thereto. Springfield: Ch. C Thomas.

— (1933), "Dyspituitarism": twenty years later. With special consideration of the pituitary adenomas. Arch. Int. Med. 51, 487—557.

— Eisenhardt, L. (1938), Meningiomas.—Their classification, regional behaviour, life history, and surgical results. Springfield: Ch. C Thomas.

Daniel, P. M., Prichard, M. L. (1958), Regeneration of the anterior pituitary after extensive infarction due to pituitary stalk section. J. Physiol. (Lond.) 143, 25P—26P.

Davidoff, L. M. (1926), Studies in acromegaly. III. The anamnesis and symptomatology in one hundred cases. Endocrinology 10, 461—483.

— (1940), Hyperpituitarism and hyopituitarism. Bull. N. Y. Acad. Med. 16, 227—243.

— Feiring, E. H. (1948), Surgical treatment of tumors of the pituitary body. Amer. J. Surg. 75, 99—136.

Deaton, P. C., Dugger, G. S. (1972), The ultrastructure of the nonadenomatous anterior lobe of the pituitary gland in man. Surg. Gynec., Obst. 135, 901—907.

Debeljuk, L., Arimura, A., Shiino, M., Rennels, E. G., Schally, A. V. (1973), Effects of chronic treatment with LH/FSH-RH in hypophysectomized pituitary-grafted male rats. Endocrinology 92, 921—930.

DeCicco, F. A., Dekker, A., Yunis, E. J. (1972), Fine structure of Crooke's hyaline change in the human pituitary gland. Arch. Path. (Chicago) 94, 65—70.

Deery, E. M. (1929), Note on calcification in pituitary adenomas. Endocrinology 13, 455—458.

De Gennes, L., Bricaire, H., Leprat, J., Vallée, B. (1963), Tumeurs hypophysaires et maladie de Cushing. A propos d'une observation personelle. Presse Méd. 71, 903—906.

Dekker, A. (1967), Pituitary basophils of the Syrian hamster: An electron microscopic investigation. Anat. Rec. 158, 351—367.

Delarue, J., Chomette, G., Pinaudeau, Y., Brocheriou, C., Auriol, M. (1964), Les métastases hypophysaires. Fréquence. Etude histopathologique. Arch. Anat. Path. (Paris) 12, 179—182.

Delthil, S., Julou, M. J. (1960), Adénome hypophysaire post-gravidique (rôle possible des oestrogènes). Bull. Soc. Ophth. Franc. 5, 336—340.

Del Vivo, E., Armenise, B., Regli, R. (1962), Varietà formali e problemi istogenetici del craniofaringioma. Arch. de Vecchi 38, 1—79.

De Virgiliis, G. (1968), Ultrastructure des cellules gonadotropes de l'adéno-hypophyse après ovarectomie. Ann. Endocr. (Paris) 29, 553—561.

— Medolesi, J., Clementi, F. (1968), Ultrastructure of growth hormone-producing cells of rat pituitary after injection of hypothalamic extract. Endocrinology 83, 1278—1284.

— Staudacher, C. (1971), Modifications de l'adéno-hypophyse après traitement à la noréthine-mestranol. Etude au microscope électronique. Ann. Endocr. (Paris) 32, 469—481.

Diepen, R. (1962), Der Hypothalamus. In: W. von Möllendorff (ed.): Handbuch der mikroskopischen Anatomie des Menschen. Vol. IV/7. Berlin-Göttingen-Heidelberg: Springer.

Dingemans, K. P. (1970), Undifferentiated cells in the mouse adenohypophysis. Congr. Internatl. El. Micr. VII, p. 563—564. Grenoble.

Dingemans, K. P., Feltkamp, C. A. (1972), Nongranulated cells in the mouse adenohypophysis. Z. Zellforsch. *124*, 387—405.

Doron, Y., Behar, A., Beller, A. J. (1965), Granular-cell myoblastoma of the neurohypophysis. J. Neurosurg. *22*, 95—99.

Dott, N. M., Bailey, P., Cushing, H. (1925), A consideration of the hypophysial adenomata. Brit. J. Surg. *13*, 314—366.

Douglas, W. H. (1970), Perchloric acid extraction of deoxiribonucleic acid from thin sections of epon-araldite-embedded material. J. Histochem. Cytochem. *18*, 510—514.

Douglas, W. W., Nagasawa, J., Schulz, R. (1971), Electron microscopic studies on the mechanism of secretion of posterior pituitary hormones and significance of microvesicles ("synaptic vesicles"): Evidence of secretion by exocytosis and formation of microvesicles as a by-product of this process. In: H. Heller, K. Lederis (eds.): Subcellular organization and function in endocrine tissues. Cambridge: Cambridge University Press.

Dubois, P. (1967), Etude au microscope électronique de la pars distalis de l'hypophyse de l'embryon humain. Bull. Ass. Anat. (Nancy) *138*, 434—441.

— (1968), Données ultrastructurales sur l'anthéhypophyse d'un embryon humain à la huitième semaine de son développement. C. R. Soc. Biol. (Paris) *162*, 689—692.

— (1970), Cytologie de l'hypophyse de bovins: Séparation des cellules somatotropes et des cellules à prolactine par immunofluorescence. Identification des cellules LH dans la pars tuberalis et la pars intermedia. Bull. Ass. Anat. (Nancy) *145*, 139—146.

— Cohere, G. (1970), Cytologie ultrastructurale du lobe antérieur et de la pars tuberalis de l'hypophyse de bovins. Bull. Ass. Anat. (Nancy) *145*, 147—157.

— Dumont, L. (1965), Observation en microscopie électronique du lobe antérieur de l'hypophyse embryonnaire humaine au troisième mois de la vie intra-utérine. C. R. Soc. Biol. (Paris) *159*, 1574—1576.

— — (1966), Nouvelles observations au microscope électronique sur l'anthéhypophyse humaine du troisième au cinquième mois du développement embryonnaire. C. R. Soc. Biol. (Paris) *160*, 2105—2108.

— Girod, C. (1969), Aspects ultrastructuraux des cellules limitant les formations colloidales dans l'anthéhypophyse du hérisson. C. R. Soc. Biol. (Paris) *163*, 1390—1393.

Duchen, L. W. (1962), The effects of ingestion of hypertonic saline on the pituitary gland in the rat: A morphological study of the pars intermedia and posterior lobe. J. Endocr. *25*, 161—168.

Duffell, D., Farber, L., Chou, S., Hartmann, J. F., Nelson, E. (1963), Electron microscopic observations on astrocytomas. Amer. J. Path. *43*, 539—554.

Duffy, W. C. (1920), Hypophysial duct tumors. A report of three cases and a fourth case of cyst of Rathke's pouch. Ann. Surg. *72*, 537—555, 725—757.

Dugger, G. S., Stratford, J. G., Bouchard, J. (1954), Necrosis of the brain following Roentgen irradiation. Amer. J. Roentgenol. *72*, 953—960.

Dumont, L., Dubois, P. (1967), Quelques aspects ultrastructuraux de l'anthéhypophyse foetale humaine. Rev. Lyon. Méd. *16*, 593—606.

Ectors, F., Danguy, A., Pasteels, J. L. (1972), Ultrastructure of organ cultures of rat hypophyses exposed to ergocornine. J. Endocr. *52*, 211—212.

Ekholm, R. (1964), Thyroid gland. In: S. M. Kurtz (ed.): Electron microscopic anatomy. New York: Academic Press.

Elfvin, L.-G. (1965), The ultrastructure of the capillary fenestrae in the adrenal medulla of the rat. J. Ultrastruct. Res. *12*, 687—704.

Elliott, R. L., Arhelger, R. B. (1966), Fine structure of a parathyroid adenoma. With special reference to annulate lamellae and septate demosomes. Arch. Path. (Chicago) *81*, 200—212.

Elwood, W. K., Bernstein, M. H. (1968), The ultrastructure of the enamel organ related to enamel formation. Amer. J. Anat. *122*, 73—94.

Endter, F., Gebauer, H. (1956), Ein einfaches Gerät zur statistischen Auswertung von mikroskopischen bzw. elektronenmikroskopischen Aufnahmen. Optik *13*, 97—101.

Eneroth, C.-M., Jacobsson, F. (1972), Große Speicheldrüsen. In: L. Diethelm, O. Olsson, F. Strnad, H. Vieten, A. Zuppinger (eds.): Handbuch der medizinischen Radiologie. Vol. 19, Part 1. Spezielle Strahlentherapie maligner Tumoren. Berlin-Heidelberg-New York: Springer.

Ennuyer, A., Cheguillaume, J. (1958), Radiothérapie transcutanée. In: G. Guiot (ed.): Adénomes hypophysaires. Paris: Masson.

Epstein, J. A., Epstein, B. S., Molho, L., Zimmerman, H. M. (1964), Carcinoma of the pituitary gland with metastases of the spinal cord and root of the cauda equina. J. Neurosurg. *21*, 846—853.

Erdheim, J. (1904), Über Hypophysenganggeschwülste und Hirncholesteatome. S. Ber. Akad. Wiss. Wien, Math.-naturwiss. Kl., Abt. III. *113*, 537—726.

— (1910), Über das eosinophile und basophile Hypophysenadenom. Frankf. Z. Path. *4*, 70—86.

— (1926), Pathologie der Hypophysengeschwülste. Erg. Path. 21/II. 482—561.

— Stumme, E. (1909), Über die Schwangerschaftsveränderung der Hypophyse. Beitr. path. Anat. *46*, 1—132.

Erlandson, R. A., Tandler, B., Lieberman, P. H., Higinbotham, N. L. (1968), Ultrastructure of human chordoma. Cancer Res. *28*, 2115—2125.

Escourolle, E., Poirier, J. (1971), Etude en microscopie électronique des tumeurs du système nerveux. Neurochirurgie *17*, Suppl. 1, 25—49.

Evans, H. M., Sparks, L. L., Dixon, J. S. (1966), The physiology and chemistry of adrenocorticotrophin. In: G. W. Harris, B. T. Donovan (eds.): The pituitary gland. Vol. 1. London: Butterworths.

Ewing, J. (1940), Neoplastic diseases. 4th ed., p. 247—248. Philadelphia: W. B. Saunders.

Ezrin, C., Murray, S. (1963), The cells of the human adenohypophysis in pregnancy, thyroid disease and adrenal cortical disorders. In: J. Benoit, C. Da Lage (eds.): Cytologie de l'adénohypophyse. Paris: Editions du Centre National de la Recherche Scientifique.

Farquhar, M. G. (1957), "Corticotrophs" of the rat adenohypophysis as revealed by electron microscopy. Anat. Rec. *127*, 291 (abstr.).

— (1961a), Fine structure and function in capillaries of the anterior pituitary gland. Angiology *12*, 270—292.

— (1961b), Origin and fate of secretory granules in cells of the anterior pituitary gland. Trans. N. Y. Acad. Sci. *23*, 346—351.

Farquhar, M. G. (1969), Lysosomes function in regulating secretion: disposal of secretory granules in cells of the anterior pituitary gland. In: J. T. Dingle, H. B. Fell (eds.): Lysosomes in Biology and Pathology. Vol. 2, pp. 462—482. Amsterdam: North-Holland Publishing Co.

— (1971), Processing of secretory products by cells of the anterior pituitary gland. In: H. Heller, K. Lederis (eds.): Subcellular organization and function in endocrine tissues. Cambridge: Cambridge University Press.

— Palade, G. E. (1963), Junctional complexes in various epithelia. J. Cell Biol. 17, 375—412.

— Rinehart, J. F. (1954a), Electron microscopic studies of the anterior pituitary gland of castrate rats. Endocrinology 54, 516—541.

— — (1954b), Cytologic alterations in the anterior pituitary gland following thyreoidectomy: an electron microscope study. Endocrinology 55, 857—876.

— — (1955), Further evidence for the existence of two types of gonadotrophs in the anterior pituitary of the rat. Anat. Rec. 121, 394 (abstr.).

— Wellings, S. R. (1957), Electron microscopic evidence suggesting secretory granule formation within the Golgi apparatus. J. Biophys. Biochem. Cytol. 3, 319—322.

Fasske, E. (1958), Über einen primär malignen Hypophysentumor bei einem Säugling. Zbl. allg. Path. 98, 281—286.

Fawcett, D. W., Long, J. A., Jones, A. L. (1969), The ultrastructure of endocrine glands. Recent Progr. Hormone Res. 25, 315—368.

Fechner, R. E., Bentinck, B. R. (1973), Ultrastructure of bronchial oncocytoma. Cancer 31, 1451—1457.

Feiring, E. H., Davidoff, L. M., Zimmerman, H. M. (1953), Primary carcinoma of the pituitary. J. Neuropath. Exp. Neurol. 12, 205—223.

Feldman, P. S., Horvath, E., Kovacs, K. (1972), Ultrastructure of three Hürthle cell tumors of the thyroid. Cancer 30, 1279—1285.

Feltkamp, C. A. (1970), Regulation of activity and number of LTH-cells, p. 567—568. Grenoble: Congr. Internatl. El. Micr. VII.

Fernandez-Moràn, H., Luft, R. (1949), Submicroscopic cytoplasmic granules in the anterior lobe cells of the rat hypophysis as revealed by electron microscopy. Acta Endocr. (Kobenhavn) 2, 199—211.

Fisher, E. R., Wechsler, H. (1962), Granular cell myoblastoma— a misnomer. Electron microscopic and histochemical evidence concerning its Schwann cell derivation and nature (granular cell Schwannoma). Cancer 15, 936—954.

Foncin, J. F. (1966), Etudes sur l'hypophyse humaine au microscope électronique. Path. Biol. 14, 893—902.

— (1971), Morphologie ultra-structurale de l'hypophyse humaine. Neurochirurgie 17, Suppl. 1, 10—24.

— Le Beau, J. (1963), Etude en microscopie optique et électronique d'une tumeur hypophysaire à fonction adrénocorticotrope. C. R. Soc. Biol. (Paris) 157, 249—252.

— — (1964), Identification au microscope électronique des cellules adrénocorticotropes de l'hypophyse humaine. C. R. Soc. Biol. (Paris) 158, 2276—2279.

— — (1966), Cellules de castration et cellules FSH dans l'hypophyse humaine vues au microscope électronique. J. Microscopie 5, 523—526.

Foncin, J. F., Le Beau, J., Billet, R. (1972), A propos des tumeurs hypophysaires extensives à sécrétion corticotrope (étude ultrastructurale). Ann. Endocr. (Paris) *33*, 449—454.

Forbes, A. P., Henneman, P. H., Griswald, G. C., Albright, F. (1954), A syndrome characterized by galactorrhea, amenorrhea and low urinary FSH: comparison with acromegaly and normal lactation. J. Clin. Endocr. *14*, 265—271.

Foster, C. L. (1956), Some observations upon the cytology of the pars distalis of surgically removed human pituitary. J. Micr. Sci. *97*, 379—391.

— (1971), Relationship between ultrastructure and function in the adenohypophysis of the rabbit. In: H. Heller, K. Lederis (eds.): Sucellular organization and function in endocrine tissues. Cambridge: Cambridge University Press.

Frazier, C. H. (1930), A series of pituitary pictures. Commentaries on the pathologic, clinical and therapeutic aspects. Arch. Neurol. Psych. (Chicago) *23*, 656—695.

— Alpers, B. J. (1931), Adamantinoma of the craniopharyngeal duct. Arch. Neurol. Psych. (Chicago) *26*, 905—965.

Friederici, H. H. R. (1968), The tridimensional ultrastructure of fenestrated capillaries. J. Ultrastruct. Res. *23*, 444—456.

Friedman, I., Harrison, D. F. N., Bird, E. S. (1962), The fine structure of chordoma with particular reference to the physaliphorous cell. J. Clin. Path. *15*, 116—125.

Frobes, W. (1947), Carcinoma of the pituitary gland with metastases to the liver in a case of Cushing's syndrome. J. Path. Bact. *59*, 137—144.

Fukuda, T. (1973), Agranular stellate cells (so-called follicular cells) in human fetal and adult adenohypophysis and in pituitary adenoma. Virchow's Arch. Abt. A, Path. Anat. *359*, 19—30.

Fust, J. A., Custer, R. P. (1948), Granular cell "myoblastomas" and granular cell neurofribomas: separation of neurogenous tumors from the myoblastoma group. Amer. J. Path. *24*, 647.

— — (1949), On the neurogenesis of the so-called granular cell myoblastoma. Amer. J. Clin. Path. *19*, 522—535.

Gamboa, L. G. (1955), Malignant granular-cell myoblastoma. Arch. Path. (Chicago) *60*, 663—668.

Garancis, J. C., Komorowski, R. A., Kuzma, J. F. (1970), Granular cell myoblastoma. Cancer *25*, 542—550.

German, W. J., Flanigan, S. (1964), Pituitary adenomas: A followup study of the Cushing series. Clin. Neurosurg. *10*, 72—81.

Gessaga, E. C., Mair, W. G. P., Grant, D. N. (1973), Ultrastructure of a sacrococcygeal chordoma. Acta Neuropath. (Berl.) *25*, 27—35.

Ghatak, N. R., Hirano, A., Zimmerman, H. M. (1971), Ultrastructure of a craniopharyngeoma. Cancer *27*, 1465—1475.

Gilbert-Dreyfus, Zara, M. (1951), La cellule de Crooke: cellule réactionelle au cours de l'hypercorticisme. Bull. Mém. Soc. Méd. Hôp. Paris *67*, 660—663.

Gilmour, M. D. (1932), Carcinoma of the pituitary gland with abdominal metastases. J. Path. Bact. *35*, 265—269.

Giok, K. H. (1961), An experimental study of pituitary tumours. Genesis, cytology and hormone content. Berlin-Göttingen-Heidelberg: Springer.

Girod, C., Dubois, P. (1965), Etude ultrastructurale des cellules gonado-
trophes antéhypophysaires, chez le Hamster doré (Mesocricetus auratus
Waterh.). J. Ultrastruct. Res. *13*, 212—232.

Glazer, N., Hauser, H., Slade, H. (1956), Granular cell tumor of the neurohypophysis. Amer. J. Roentgenol. *76*, 324—326.

Goldberg, G. M., Eshbaugh, D. E. (1960), Squamous cell nests of the pituitary
gland as related to the origin of craniopharyngiomas. Arch. Path.
(Chicago) *70*, 293—299.

Goldberg, M. B., Sheline, G. E., Malamud, N. (1963), Malignant intracranial neoplasms following radiation therapy for acromegaly. Radiology
80, 465—470.

Golden, A., Bondy, P. K., Sheldon, W. H. (1950), Pituitary basophile
hyperplasia and Crooke's hyaline changes in man after ACTH therapy.
Proc. Soc. Exp. Biol. Med. *74*, 455—458.

Gon, F. (1965), Calcifying epithelial odontogenic tumor.—Report of a case
and a study of its histogenesis. Brit. J. Cancer *19*, 39—50.

Gordy, P. D., Peet, M. M., Kahn, E. A. (1949), The surgery of craniopharyngiomas. J. Neurosurg. *6*, 503—517.

Gorlin, R. J., Chaudhry, A. P., Pindborg, J. J. (1961), Odontogenic tumors.
Classification, histopathology, and clinical behaviour in man and do-
mesticated animals. Cancer *14*, 73—101.

Graf, C. J., Blinderman, E. E., Terplan, K. L. (1962), Pituitary carcinoma
in a child with distant metastases. J. Neurosurg. *19*, 254—259.

Grant, F. C. (1948), Surgical experience with tumors of the pituitary gland.
J. A. M. A. *136*, 668—671.

Gray, E. G. (1964), Tissue of the central nervous system. In: S. M. Kurtz
(ed.): Electron microscopic anatomy, p. 369—417. New York: Academic
Press.

Gray, S. H., Gruenfeld, G. E. (1937), Myoblastoma. Amer. J. Cancer *30*,
699—708.

Green, J. D. (1966a), Electron microscopy of the anterior pituitary. In:
G. W. Harris, B. T. Donovan (eds.): The pituitary gland. Vol. 1. London: Butterworths.

— (1966b), Microanatomical aspects of the formation of neurohypophysial
hormones and neurosecretion. In: G. W. Harris, B. T. Donovan (eds.):
The pituitary gland. Vol. 3. London: Butterworths.

— Van Breemen, V. L. (1955), Electron microscopy of the pituitary and
observations on neurosecretion. Amer. J. Anat. *97*, 177—227.

Gullotta, F. (1973), Personal communication.

— Fliedner, E. (1972), Spongioblastomas, astrocytomas and Rosenthal
fibers. Ultrastructural, tissue culture and enzyme histochemical investigations. Acta Neuropath. (Berl.) *22*, 68—78.

— Klein, H. (1973), La microscopia elettronica nella diagnostica tumorale.
Neoplasia atipica della regione ipofisaria identificata con l'ultramicro-
scopio (,,carcinoma" dell'ipofisi). Pathologica *65*, 353—355.

Gusek, W. (1962), Vergleichende licht- und elektronenmikroskopische
Untersuchungen menschlicher Hypophysenadenome bei Akromegalie.
Endokrinologie *42*, 257—283.

Guyda, H., Robert, F., Colle, E., Hardy, J. (1973), Histologic, ultrastructural, and hormonal characterization of a pituitary tumor secreting
both hGH and prolactin. J. Clin. Endocrinol. Metab. *36*, 531—547.

Györkey, F., Min, K.-W., Sincovics, J. G., Györkey, P. (1969), Systemic lupus erythematosus and myxovirus. New Engl. J. Med. *280*, 333.
— Sinkovics, J. G., Györkey, P. (1971), Electron microscopic observations on structure resembling myxovirus in human sarcomas. Cancer *27*, 1449—1454.
Hachmeister, U. (1973a), Ultrastructural aspects of pituitary tumors. In: H. Kuhlendahl, M. Brock, D. Le Vay, T. J. Weston (eds.): Modern aspects of neurosurgery. Vol. 4.—Proceedings of the German society for neurosurgery. Amsterdam: Excerpta Medica.
— (1973b), Ultrastructural aspects of endocrine activity in "chromophobic" pituitary adenomas. Acta endocr. (Kbh.). Suppl. *173*, 153.
— Fahlbusch, R., Werder, K. v. (1972), Ultrastructural identity of pituitary adenoma cells in Forbes-Albright syndrome and of adenohypophyseal pregnancy cells. Acta endocr. (Kbh.) Suppl. *159*, 42 (abstr.).
— Wiegelmann, W., Solbach, H. G. (1971), Ultrastructure and hormone distribution of the human corticotropic anterior pituitary cell under normal condition, in corticotropic adenoma and in exogenous hypercortisolism. Acta endocr. (Kbh.) Suppl. *152*, 90 (abstr.).
Hägerstrand, I., Schönebeck, J. (1969), Metastases to the pituitary gland. Acta Path. Microbiol. Scand. *75*, 64—70.
Halmi, N. S., McCormick, W. F., Decker, D. A. (1971), The natural history of hyalinization of ACTH-MSH cells in man. Arch. Path. (Chicago) *91*, 318—326.
Hamperl, H. (1931), Onkocyten und Geschwülste der Speicheldrüsen. Virchow's Arch. *282*, 724—736.
— (1933), Über besondere Zellen in alternden Mundspeicheldrüsen (Onkocyten) und ihre Beziehungen zu den Adenolymphomen und Adenomen. Virchow's Arch. *291*, 704—705.
— (1937), Über das Vorkommen von Onkocyten in verschiedenen Organen und ihren Geschwülsten. Virchow's Arch. *298*, 327—375.
— (1950), Oncocytes and the so-called Hürthle-cell tumor. Arch. Path. (Chicago) *49*, 563—567.
— (1962a), Onkocyten und Onkocytome. Virchow's Arch. *335*, 452—483.
— (1962b), Benign and malignant oncocytoma. Cancer *15*, 1019—1027.
Harland, W. A. (1956), Granular cell myoblastoma of the hypophyseal stalk. Cancer *6*, 1134—1138.
Hastrup, J. (1966), Chromophobe adenoma of the pituitary with extensive calcifications. Acta Neuropath. (Berl.) *6*, 98—100.
Heath, E. (1970), Cytology of the pars anterior of the bovine adenohypophysis. Amer. J. Anat. *127*, 131—157.
Hedinger, C. E., Farquhar, M. G. (1957), Elektronenmikroskopische Untersuchungen von zwei Typen acidophiler Hypophysenvorderlappenzellen bei der Ratte. Schweiz. Z. path. Bakt. *20*, 766—768.
Heinemann, P., Ljunggren, J.-G., Löwhagen, T., Hjern, B. (1973), Oxyphilic adenoma of the human thyroid. Cancer *31*, 246—254.
Heimbach, S. B. (1959), Follow-up studies on 105 cases of verified chromophobe and acidophile pituitary adenomata after treatment by transfrontal operation and X-ray irradiation. Acta Neurochir. (Wien) *7*, 101—155.
Henderson, W. R. (1939), The pituitary adenomata. A follow-up study of the surgical results in 338 cases (Dr. Harvey Cushing's series). Brit. J. Surg. *26*, 811—921.

Herlant, M. (1960), Etude critique de deux techniques nouvelles destinées à mettre en évidence les différentes catégories cellulaires présentes dans la glande pituitaire. Bull. Micr. Appl. *10*, 37—44.

— (1963), Apport de la microscopie électronique à l'étude du lobe antérieur de l'hypophyse. In: J. Benoit, C. Da Lage (eds.): Cytologie de l'adénohypophyse. Paris: Editions du Centre National de la Recherche Scientifique.

— (1964), The cells of the adenohypophysis and their functional significance. Int. Rev. Cytol. *17*, 299—382.

— (1965), Present state of knowledge concerning the cytology of the anterior lobe of the hypophysis. Proc. 2nd, Int. Congr. Endocrinol. 1964, p. 468. Amsterdam: Excerpta Medica.

— Decourt, J. (1964), Identification des cellules corticotropes dans un adénome hypophysaire ayant déterminé une maladie de Cushing. Sem. Hôp. Paris *40*, 1426—1431.

— Klasterky, J. (1963), Etude au microscope électronique des cellules corticotropes de l'hypophyse. C. R. Acad. Sci. (Paris) *256*, 2709—2711.

— Laine, E., Fossati, P., Linquette, M. (1965), Syndrome aménorrhée-galactorrhée par adénome hypophysaire à cellules à prolactine. Ann. Endocr. (Paris) *26*, 65—71.

Herndon, R. M., Rubinstein, L. J. (1968), Light and electron microscopy observations on the development of viral particles in the inclusions of Dawson's encephalitis (subacute sclerosing panencephalitis). Neurology (Minneap.) *18*, 8—20.

Hirano, A. (1971), Electron microscopy in neuropathology. Progr. Neuropath. *1*, 1—61.

— Tomiyasu, U., Zimmerman, H. M. (1972), The fine structure of blood vessels in chromophobe adenoma. Acta Neuropath. (Berl.) *22*, 200—207.

Hoff, J. T., Patterson, R. H. (1972), Craniopharyngiomas in children and adults. J. Neurosurg. *36*, 299—302.

Holmes, R. L. (1964), Comparative observations on inclusions in nerve fibres of the mammalian neurohypophysis. Z. Zellforsch. *64*, 474—492.

Horsley, V. (1906), On the technique of operations on the central nervous system. Brit. Med. J. *II*, 411—423.

Hossmann, K.-A., Wechsler, W. (1965), Zur Feinstruktur menschlicher Spongioblastome. Dtsch. Z. Nervenheilk. *187*, 327—351.

— — (1967), Elektronenmikroskopie kindlicher Hirngeschwülste. In: H. Kraus, M. Sunder-Plassmann (eds.), Pädiatrische Neurochirurgie, pp. 77—88. Wien: Ber. 1. Europ. Kongr. 1967.

Houck, W. A., Olson, K. B., Horton, J. (1970), Clinical features of tumor metastasis to the pituitary. Cancer *26*, 656—659.

Howe, A., Maxwell, D. S. (1968), Electron microscopy of the pars intermedia of the pituitary gland in the rat. Gen. Comp. Endocr. *11*, 169—185.

Hübner, G., Klein, H. J., Schummelfeder, N. (1965), Zur Ultrastruktur der Oncocytome. Klin. Wschr. *43*, 798—800.

— Paulussen, F., Kleinsasser, O. (1967), Zur Feinstruktur und Genese der Onkocyten. Virchow's Arch. *343*, 34—50.

Hunter, I. J. (1955), Squamous metaplasia of cells of the anterior pituitary gland. J. Path. Bact. *69*, 141—145.

Hürthle, K. (1894), Beitrag zur Kenntnis des Sekretionsvorganges in der Schilddrüse. Pflügers Arch. ges. Physiol. *56*, 1—44.

Husten, K. (1923), Über zwei Beobachtungen von Hypophysengangstumoren. Virchow's Arch. *242*, 222—238.

Hymer, W. C., Kraicer, J., Bencosme, S. A., Haskill, J. S. (1972), Separation of somatotrophs from the rat adenohypophysis by velocity and density gradient centrifugation. Proc. Soc. Exp. Biol. Med. *141*, 966—973.

— Evans, W. H., Kraicer, J., Mastro, A., Davis, J., Griswold, E. (1973), Enrichment of cell types from the rat adenohypophysis by sedimentation at unit gravity. Endocrinology *92*, 275—287.

Jackson, I. M. D. (1965), Hyperthyroidism in a patient with a pituitary chromophobe adenoma. J. Clin. Endocr. Metab. *25*, 491—494.

Jayatilaka, A. D. P. (1965), An electron microscopic study of sheep arachnoid granulations. J. Anat. (Lond.) *99*, 635—649.

Jefferson, G. (1954), The invasive adenomas of the anterior pituitary. Liverpool: University Press of Liverpool.

Jenevein, E. P. (1964), A neurohypophyseal tumor originating from pituicytes. Amer. J. Clin. Path. *41*, 522—526.

Jenis, E. H., Knieser, M. R., Rothouse, P. A., Jensen, G. E., Scott, R. M. (1973), Subacute sclerosing panencephalitis. Immunoultrastructural localization of measles-virus antigen. Arch. Path. (Chicago) *95*, 81—89.

Jenson, A. B., Spjut, H. J., Smith, M. N., Rapp, F. (1971), Intracellular branched tubular structures in osteosarcoma. An ultrastructural and serological study. Cancer *27*, 1440—1448.

Iliescu, V. (1969), Tumora granulara a lobului posterior al hipofizei. (Prezentare de caz). Stud. Cercet. Endocrinol. *20*, 259—263.

Ito, A., Furth, J., Moy, P. (1972), Growth hormone-secreting variants of a mamotropic tumor. Cancer Res. *32*, 48—56.

Justin-Besançon, L., Péquignot, H., Grivaux, M., De Pailieret, F. (1959), Un cas de myxoedème congénital avec adénome hypophysaire. Sem. Hôp. Paris *35*, 177—182.

Kagayama, M. (1965), The follicular cell in the pars distalis of the dog pituitary gland: An electron microscope study. Endocrinology *77*, 1053—1060.

Kalnins, V., Rossi, E. (1965), Odontogenic craniopharyngioma. Cancer *18*, 899—906.

Kappeler, R. (1959), Hyperthyreose und Panhypopituitarismus im Verlauf eines chromophoben Adenoms der Hypophyse. Schweiz. med. Wschr. *89*, 367—369.

Kawarai, Y., Nakane, P. K. (1970), Localization of tissue antigens on the ultrathin sections with peroxidase-labeled antibody method. J. Histochem. Cytochem. *18*, 161—166.

Kay, S., Schatzki, P. F. (1972), Ultratructural observations of a chordoma arising in the clivus. Human Path. *3*, 403—413.

— Still, J. S. (1973), Electron microscopic observations on a parotid oncocytoma. Arch. Path. (Chicago) *96*, 186—188.

Kepeler, E. J. (1945), The relationship of "Crooke's changes" in the basophilic cells of the anterior pituitary body to Cushing's syndrome (pituitary basophilism). J. Clin. Endocr. *5*, 70—75.

Kepes, J. (1961), Electron microscopic studies of meningiomas. Amer. J. Path. *39*, 499—510.

Kernohan, J. W., Sayre, G. P. (1956), Tumors of the pituitary gland and infundibulum. Atlas of tumor pathology, section X, fascicle 36. Washington: Armed Forces Institute of Pathology.

Kersting, G. (1961), Die Gewebszüchtung menschlicher Hirngeschwülste. Berlin-Göttingen-Heidelberg: Springer.

Kilby, R. A., Bennett, W. A., Sprague, R. G. (1957), Anterior pituitary glands in patients treated with cortisone and corticotropin. Amer. J. Path. *33*, 155—173.

King, A. B. (1951), The diagnosis of carcinoma of the pituitary gland. Bull. Johns Hopkins Hosp. *89*, 339—353.

Kirsch, W. M., Nakane, P. K. (1973), A histochemical examination of pituitary adenomas with enzyme-labelled antibodies. In: R. Carrea, S. Ishii, D. Le Vay (eds.): 5th Int. Congr. Neurol. Surg. — Int. Congr. Series No. 293, p. 35. Amsterdam: Excerpta Medica.

Kiyono, H. (1926), Histopathologie der Hypophyse. Virchow's Arch. *259*, 388—465.

Klemperer, P. (1934), Myoblastoma of the striated muscle. Amer. J. Cancer *20*, 324—337.

Kobayashi, Y. (1964), Functional morphology of the pars intermedia of the rat hypophysis as revealed with the electron microscope. I. Ultra-structural changes after dehydration. Gunma Symp. Endocr. *1*, 173—181.

— (1965), Functional morphology of the pars intermedia of the rat hypophysis as revealed with the electron microscope. II. Correlation of the pars intermedia with the hypophysio-adrenal axis. Z. Zellforsch. *68*, 155—171.

Köhlmeier, W. (1944), Zur Kenntnis der metastasierenden Hypophysengeschwülste. Virchow's Arch. *312*, 26—34.

Kontchakova, M. (1936), Metastasen von Tumoren der Hypophyse, ihre pathologische Anatomie und Klinik. Sovet. Psichonevrol. *12*, 109—112. — Ref. Zbl. Ges. Neurol. *86*, 572 (1937).

Korbine, A. I., Ross, E. (1973), Granular cell myoblastomas of the pituitary region. Surg. Neurol. *1*, 275—279.

Kovacs, K. (1973), Metastatic cancer of the pituitary gland. Oncology *27*, 533—542.

— Horvath, E. (1973), Pituitary "chromophobe" adenoma composed of oncocytes. A light and electron microscopic study. Arch. Path. (Chicago) *95*, 235—239.

Kracht, J. (1957), Zur Lokalisation der Hypophysenvorderlappenhormone. Zbl. allg. Path. *97*, 24—35.

Kraus, E. J. (1923), Zur Pathologie der basophilen Zellen der Hypophyse. Zugleich ein Beitrag zur Pathologie des Morbus Basedowi und Addisoni. Virchow's Arch. *247*, 421—447.

— (1926), Die Hypophyse. In: F. Henke und O. Lubarsch (eds.): Handbuch der speziellen pathologischen Anatomie und Histologie. Vol. 8: Drüsen mit innerer Sekretion, p. 810—950. Berlin: Springer.

— (1945), Neoplastic diseases of the human hypophysis. Arch. Path. (Chicago) *39*, 343—349.

Krause, F. (1927), Bemerkungen zur Operation der Hypophysengeschwülste. Dtsch. med. Wschr. *53*, 691—694.

Krayenbühl, H., Rüttner, J. R. (1973), Röntgenspätschäden des Schläfenhirns nach Hochvoltbestrahlung maligner Tumoren des Epipharynx. Schweiz. med. Wschr. *103*, 225—231.

Krestin, D. (1932), Spontaneous lactation associated with enlargement of the pituitary. Lancet *1*, 928—930.

Krieg, A. F. (1962), Malignant granular cell myoblastoma. Arch. Path. (Chicago) *74*, 251—256.

Kuromatsu, C. (1967), The fine structure of the human pituitary chromophobe adenoma. Neurol. Medicochir. (Tokyo) *9*, 43—44.

Kurosumi, K., Matsuzawa, T., Shibasaki, S. (1961), Electron microscope studies on the fine structure of the pars nervosa and pars intermedia, and their morphological interrelation in the normal rat hypophysis. Gen. Comp. Endocr. *1*, 433—452.

— Oota, Y. (1966), Corticotrophs in the anterior pituitary glands of gonadectomized and thyroidectomized rats as revealed by electron microscopy. Endocrinology *79*, 808—814.

— — (1968), Electron microscopy of two types of gonadotrophs in the anterior pituitary gland of persistent estrus and persistent diestrus rats. Z. Zellforsch. *85*, 34—46.

Labrie, F., Gauthier, M., Pelletier, G., Borgeat, P., Lemay, A., Gouge, J.-J. (1973), Role of microtubules in basal and stimulated release of growth hormone and prolactin in rat adenohypophysis in vitro. Endocrinology *93*, 903—914.

Lampert, P. W., Davis, R. L. (1964), Delayed effects of radiation on the human central nervous system. "Early" and "late" delayed reactions. Neurology (Minneap.) *14*, 912—917.

Landolt, A. M. (1972), Die Ultrastruktur des Kraniopharyngioms. Schweiz. Arch. Neurol. Neurochir. Psychiat. *111*, 313—329.

— (1973a), Regeneration of the human pituitary. J. Neurosurg. *39*, 35—41.

— (1973b), The oncocytoma, a new histological type of pituitary adenoma. In: H. Kuhlendahl, M. Brock, D. Le Vay, T. J. Weston (eds.): Modern Aspects of Neurosurgery. Vol. 4.—Proceedings of the German Society for neurosurgery. Amsterdam: Excerpta Medica.

— (1974a), L'oncocytome, un nouveau type histologique des adénomes hypophysaires. Oto-Neuro-Ophthal. *47*, 237—252.

— (1974b), Can craniopharyngiomas be treated by radiotherapy (histologic and ultrastructural considerations)? In: K.-A. Bushe, O. Spoerri, J. Shaw (eds.): Progress in paediatric neurosurgery. Proc. 3rd Europ. Congr. Paed. Neurosurg. Göttingen, p. 232—236. Stuttgart: Hippokrates.

— Oswald, U. W. (1973), Histology and ultrastructure of an oncocytic adenoma of the human pituitary. Cancer *31*, 1099—1105.

— Ryffel, U., Hosbach, H. U., Wyler, R. (1975), Ultrastructure of tubular inclusions in endothelial cells of pituitary tumors associated with acromegaly. (In preparation.)

— Siegfried, J. (1969), Transsphenoidale, stereotaktische Elektrokoagulation der Hypophyse. Schweiz. Med. Wschr. *99*, 1296—1298.

— — (1970), Zur Behandlung maligner, metastasierender Tumoren mit der stereotaktischen transsphenoidalen Elektrokoagulation der Hypophyse. Schweiz. Med. Wschr. *100*, 1297—1306.

Lange, R. (1961), Zur Histologie und Zytologie der Glandula parathyreoidea des Menschen. Licht- und elektronenmikroskopische Untersuchungen an Epithelkörperadenomen. Z. Zellforsch. *53*, 765—828.

Langeron, L., Giard, P., Vincent, G. (1954), Myxoedème et adénomes basophiles de l'hypophyse. Bull. Acad. Nat. Méd. (Paris) *138*, 79—83.

— Croccel, L., Routier, G., Choteau, Ph. (1959), Coma myxoedémateux, involution thyroidienne et adénome éosinophile de l'hypophyse. Ann. Endocr. (Paris) *20*, 490—493.

Langhans, T. (1907), Über die epithelialen Formen der malignen Struma. Virchow's Arch. *189*, 69—188.

Laqueur, G. L. (1950), Cytological changes in human hypophysis after cortisone and ACTH treatment. Science *112*, 429—430.

Le Beau, J., Foncin, J. F. (1972), Contribution à l'étude ultrastructurale des adénomes à prolactine. Ann. Endocr. (Paris) *33*, 353—356.

Lederis, K. (1963), A preliminary report on the ultrastructure of human neurohypophysis. J. Endocrinol. *27*, 133—135.

— (1965), An electron microscopical study of the human neurohypophysis. Z. Zellforsch. *65*, 847—868.

— (1967), Electron microscopic examination of the human pituitary obtained at hypophysectomy. In: M. Dargent, C. Romieu (eds.): La chirurgie endocrinienne majeure dans le traitement du cancer du sein en phase avancée, pp. 219—222. Lyon: Simep éditions.

Le Pecqu, J.-B., Yot, P., Paoletti, C. (1964), Interaction du bromhydrate d'ethidium (BET) avec les acides nucléiques. C. R. Acad. Sci. Paris *259*, 1786—1789.

Leroux, R., Delarre, J. (1939), Sur trois cas de tumeurs à cellules granuleuses de la cavité buccale. Bull. Ass. Franç. Cancer *28*, 427—447.

Lewis, P. D., Noorden, S. van (1972), Pituitary abnormalities in acromegaly. Arch. Path. (Chicago) *94*, 119—126.

— — (1974), "Nonfunctioning" pituitary tumors. Arch. Path. (Chicago) *97*, 178—182.

Leznoff, A., Fishman, J., Goodfriend, E., McGarry, E., Beck, J., Rose, B. (1960), Localization of fluorescent antibodies to human growth hormone in human anterior pituitary glands. Proc. Soc. Exp. Biol. Med. *104*, 232—235.

Lichtensteiger, W. (1969), Cyclic variations of catecholamine content in hypothalamic nerve cells during the estrous cycle of the rat, with a concomitant study of the substantia nigra. J. Pharmacol. Exp. Ther. *165*, 204—215.

Lichtenstein, L. (1972), Bone tumors. 4th ed. St. Louis: Mosby.

Lima, A., Antunes, I., Tome, F. (1960), Pituicytoma or granular-cell myoblastoma of the pituitary gland. Report of a case. J. Neurosurg. *17*, 778—782.

Lindgren, E., Di Chiro, G. (1951), Sprasellar tumors with calcification. Acta Radiol. (Stockholm) *36*, 173—195.

Lindholm, J., Rasmussen, P., Korsgaard, O. (1969), Chromophobe adenomas of the pituitary gland in Cushing's disease. Acta Endocr. (Kobenhavn) *62*, 647—652.

Linquette, M., Herlant, M., Laine, E., Fossati, P., Dupont-Lecompte, J. (1967), Adénome à prolactine chez une fille dont la mère était porteuse d'un adénome hypophysaire avec aménorrhée-galactorrhée. Ann. Endocr. (Paris) *28*, 773—780.

— — Fossati, P., May, J.-P., Decoulx, M., Fourlinnie, J. C. (1969), Adénome hypophysaire à cellules thryéotropes avec hyperthyreoidie. Ann. Endocr. (Paris) *30*, 731—740.

Liss, L., Kahn, E. A. (1958), Pituicytoma, tumor of the sella turcica: a clinicopathological study. J. Neurosurg. *15*, 481—488.

Lloyd, R. V., McShan, W. H. (1973), Study of rar anterior pituitary cells separated by velocity sedimentation at unit gravity. Endocrinology *92*, 1639—1651.

Löffler, E. (1929), Über ortsfremde Zellen und Geschwülste im Hinterlappen und im Stil der Hypophyse. Virchow's Arch. *274*, 326—349.

Long, D. M. (1973), Vascular ultrastructure in human meningiomas and schwannomas. J. Neurosurg. *38*, 409—419.

Love, J. G., Marshall, T. M. (1950), Craniopharyngiomas (pituitary adamantinomas). Surg. Gynec. Obst. *90*, 591—601.

Luft, J. H. (1973), Embedding media—old and new. In: J. K. Kohler (ed.): Advanced techniques in biological electron microscopy, p. 1—34. Berlin-Heidelberg-New York: Springer.

Luft, R., Ikkos, R. D., Palmieri, G., Ernster, L., Afzelius, B. (1962), A case of severe hypermetabolism of nonthyroid origin with a defect in the maintenance of mitochondrial respiratory control: a correlated clinical, biochemical, and morphological study. J. Clin. Invest. *41*, 1776—1804.

Lumsden, C. E. (1971), The study by tissue culture of tumours of the nervous system. In: D. S. Russell, L. J. Rubinstein: Pathology of tumours of the nervous system. London: E. Arnold.

Luse, S. A. (1960), Electron microscopic studies of brain tumors. Neurology (Minneap.) *10*, 881—905.

— (1961), Ultrastructural characteristics of normal and neoplastic cells. Progr. Exp. Tumor Res. *2*, 1—35.

— (1962), Electron microscopy of brain tumors. In: W. S. Fields, P. C. Sharkey (eds.): The biology and treatment of intracranial tumors. Springfield: Ch. C Thomas.

— Kernohan, J. W. (1955 a), Granular-cell tumors of the stalk and posterior lobe of the pituitary gland. Cancer *8*, 616—622.

— — (1955 b), Squamous-cell nests of the pituitary gland. Cancer *8*, 623—628.

Lüthy, F., Klingler, M. (1951), Der Tumorettentumor des Hypophysenhinterlappens. Schweiz. Z. allg. Path. *14*, 721—729.

Mackay, B., Ibanec, M. L., Ayala, A. G., Tobelman, W. T. (1973), Pathology of pituitary tumors. In: Endocrine and nonendocrine hormone-producing tumors. Proc. 16th Annual. Clin. Conf. on Cancer 1971, Houston, Texas. Chicago: Year Book Medical Publishers.

Mackenzie, D. H. (1967), Malignant granular cell myoblastoma. J. Clin. Path. *20*, 739—742.

Madonick, M. J., Rubinstein, L. J., Dasco, R. M., Ribner, H. (1963), Chromophobe adenoma of the pituitary gland with subarachnoid metastases. Neurology (Minneap.) *13*, 836—840.

Mainwaring, A. R., Ahmed, A., Hopkinson, J. M., Anderson, P. (1971), A clinical and electron microscopic study of a calcifying epithelial odontogenic tumour. J. Clin. Path. *24*, 152—158.

Markesbery, W. R., Duffy, P. E., Cowen, D. (1973), Granular cell tumors of the central nervous system. J. Neuropath. Exp. Neurol. *23*, 92—109.

Marks, V. (1959), Cushing's syndrome occurring with pituitary chromophobe tumors. Acta Endocr. (Kobenhavn) *32*, 527—535.

Marshall, J. M. (1951), Localization of adrenocorticotrophic hormone by histochemical and immunochemical methods. J. Exp. Med. *94*, 21—30.

Martins, A. N., Hayes, G. J., Kempe, L. G. (1965), Invasive pituitary adenomas. J. Neurosurg. *22*, 268—276.

McCann, S. M., Porter, J. C. (1969), Hypothalamic pituitary stimulating and inhibiting hormones. Physiol. Rev. *49*, 240—284.

McCormick, W. F., Halmi, N. S. (1971), Absence of chromophobe adenomas from a large series of pituitary tumors. Arch. Path. (Chicago) *92*, 231—238.

McLean, A. J. (1936), Pituitary tumors. In: O. Bumke und O. Foerster (eds.): Handbuch der Neurologie. Vol. 14, p. 242—285. Berlin: Springer.

McPhie, J. L., Beck, J. S. (1973), The histological features and human growth hormone content of the pharyngeal pituitary gland in normal and endocrinologically-disturbed patients. Clin. Endocr. *2*, 157—173.

McShan, W. H. (1956), Ultrastructure and function of the anterior pituitary gland. Proc. 2nd Int. Congr. Endocrinol., p. 382 (1964). Amsterdam: Excerpta Med. Found.

Melnyck, C. S., Greer, M. A. (1965), Functional pituitary tumor in an adult possibly secondary to long-standing myxoedema. J. Clin. Endocr. Metab. *25*, 761—766.

Meredith, J. M., Kay, S., Bosher, L. H. (1958), Case of granular cell myoblastoma (organoid type) involving arm, lung and brain with twenty years' survival. J. Thor. Surg. *35*, 80—90.

Michard, J.-P. (1958), Endocrinologie. In: G. Guiot (ed.): Adénomes hypophysaires — Rapport présenté à la réunion annuelle de la société de neuro-chirurgie de langue française. Paris: Masson.

Mincer, H. M., McGinnis, J. P. (1972), Ultrastructure of three histologic variants of the ameloblastoma. Cancer *30*, 1036—1045.

Mink, L. M., Hackel, D. B., Yuksel, A. (1955), Identical granular cells in nodules and tumor of the neurohypophysis. Lab. Invest. *4*, 18—26.

Mirouze, J., Jaffiol, C., Mary, P., Baldet, P., Monnier, L. (1969), Deux syndromes originaux « Amenorrhée-Galactorrhée » par tumeur hypophysaire. Discussion anatomo-clinique. Etude ultrastructurale de l'un d'eux. Ann. Endocr. (Paris) *30*, 810—821.

Moberg, A. (1959), A case of pituitary chromophobe adenoma with metastases in the heart. Acta Path. Microbiol. Scand. *45*, 243—249.

Moe, H., Clausen, F., Philipsen, H. P. (1961), The ultrastructure of a simple ameloblastoma. Acta Path. Microbiol. Scand. *52*, 140—154.

Montandon, A. (1957), Quantitative und qualitative Zellveränderungen im Hypophysenvorderlappen bei therapeutischem Hypercorticismus. Virchow's Arch. *330*, 629—650.

Montgomery, D. A. D. (1964), Pituitary tumors in Cushing's syndrome. Clin. Neurosurg. *10*, 169—187.

— Welbourn, R. B., McCaughey, W. T. E., Gleadhill, C. A. (1959), Pituitary tumors manifested after adrenalectomy for Cushing's syndrome. Lancet *2*, 707—710.

Moolden, S. E., Silver, A. M., Mihalyfi, M. (1973), Self-propagating cytotoxic agent in systemic lupus erythematosus. Amer. J. Clin. Path. *60*, 123.

Moriarty, G. C., Halmi, N. S. (1972), Electron microscopic study of the adrenocorticotropin-producing cell with the use of unlabelled antibody and the soluble peroxidase complex. J. Histochem. Cytochem. *20*, 590—603.

— Moriarty, C. M., Sternberger, L. A. (1973), Ultrastructural immunochemistry with unlabeled antibodies and the peroxidase-antiperoxidase complex. J. Histochem. Cytochem. *21*, 825—833.

Mornex, R., Tommasi, M., Cure, M., Farcot, J., Orgiazzi, J., Rousset, B. (1972), Hyperthyroidie associée à un hypopituitarisme au cours de l'évolution d'une tumeur hypophysaire sécrétant TSH. Ann. Endocr. (Paris) *33*, 390—396.

Moscovic, E. A., Azar, H. A. (1967), Multiple granular cell tumors ("myoblastomas"). Case report with electron microscopic observations and review of the literature. Cancer *20*, 2032—2047.

Mugnaini, E., Walberg, F. (1964), Ultrastructure of neuroglia. Erg. Anat. Entwgesch. *37*, 194—236.

Mundinger, F., Riechert, T. (1967), Hypophysentumoren — Hypophysektomie. Klinik, Therapie, Ergebnisse. Stuttgart: Thieme.

Munger, B. L. (1958), A light and electron microscopic study of cellular differentiation in the pancreatic islets of the mouse. Amer. J. Anat. *103*, 275—311.

Murad, T. M., Murthy, M. S. N. (1970), Ultrastructure of a chordoma. Cancer *25*, 1204—1215.

Murphy, G. H., Dockerty, M. D., Broders, A. C. (1949), Myoblastoma. Amer. J. Path. *25*, 1157—1182.

Murray, M. R. (1951), Cultural characteristics of three granular-cell myoblastomas. Cancer *4*, 857—865.

Nakane, P. K. (1968), Simultaneous localization of multiple tissue antigens utilizing the peroxidase-labeled antibody method: a study on pituitary glands of the rat. J. Histochem. Cytochem. *16*, 557—560.

— (1970), Classification of anterior pituitary cell types with immunoenzyme histochemistry. J. Histochem. Cytochem. *18*, 9—20.

— (1971), Application of peroxidase-labelled antibodies to the intracellular localization of hormones. Acta. Endocr. (Kobenhavn) Suppl. *153*, 190—204.

— Pierce, G. B. (1966), Enzyme-labeled antibodies: preparation and application for localization of antigens. J. Histochem. Cytochem. *14*, 929—931.

— — (1967), Enzyme-labeled antibodies for light and electron microscopic localization of tissue antigen. J. Cell. Biol. *33*, 307—318.

Nakayama, I., Nickerson, P. A., Skelton, F. S. (1969), An ultrastructural study of the adenocorticotropic hormone-secreting cell in the rat adenohypophysis during adrenalcortical regeneration. Lab. Invest. *21*, 169—178.

Napolitano, L., Kyle, R., Fisher, E. R. (1964), Ultrastructure of meningiomas and the derivation and nature of their cellular components. Cancer *17*, 233—241.

Nayak, R., McGarry, E. E., Beck, J. C. (1968), Site of prolactin in the pituitary gland, as studied by immunofluorescence. Endocrinology *83*, 731—736.

Nelson, D. H., Meakin, J. W., Dealy, J. B., Matson, D. D., Emerson, K., Thorn, G. W. (1958), ACTH-Producing tumor of the pituitary gland. New Engl. J. Med. *259*, 161—164.

— Sprunt, J. G. (1964), Pituitary tumors post adrenalectomy for Cushing's syndrome. Proc. 2nd Intern. Congr. Endocr., p. 1053. London.

Nelson, W. O. (1941), The occurrence of hypophyseal tumors in rats under treatment with diethyl-stilboestrol. Amer. J. Physiol. *133*, P 398 (abstr.).

Newton, T. H., Burhenne, H. J., Palubinskas, A. J. (1962), Primary carcinoma of the pituitary. Amer. J. Roentgenol. *87*, 110—120.

Norris, F. H., Aguilar, M. J., Harmann, C. E. (1972), Visus-like particles in a case of vasculitis with brain tumor. Arch. Neurol. (Chicago) *26*, 212—217.

Northfield, D. W. (1957), Rathke-pouch tumors. Brain *80*, 293—323.

Norton, W. L. (1969), Endothelial inclusions in active lesions of systemic lupus erythematosus. J. Lab. Clin. Med. *74*, 369—379.

Nyhan, W. L., Green, M. (1964), Hyperthyroidism in a patient with a pituitary adenoma. J. Pediat. *65*, 583—589.

Nyström, S. H. (1965), A study of supratentorial meningiomas. With special reference to gross and fine structure. Acta Path. Microbiol. Scand. (Suppl.) *176*, 1—90.

— (1973), Basic studies on neurosurgical target tissues. Helsinki: Vammala.

Odland, G. F., Reed, T. H. (1967), Epidermis. In: A. S. Zelickson (ed.): Ultrastructure of the normal and abnormal skin. Philadelphia: Lea & Febiger.

Oliva, H., Navarro, V., Obrador, S. (1966), Microscopía electrónica de los adenomas cromófobos de la hipófisis. Acta Neurochir. (Wien) *14*, 141—153.

Olivier, L., Porcile, E., Brye, C., Racadot, J. (1965), Etude de quelques adénomes hypophysaires che l'homme en microscopie électronique. Bull. Assoc. Anat. (Nancy) *127*, 1258—1265.

— Vila-Porcile, E., Brye, C., Nouet, J. C. (1971), Les cellules folliculaires du lobe antérieur de l'adénohypophyse de chat adulte. Bull. Ass. Anat. (Nancy) *152*, 814—815.

— — Peillon, F., Racadot, J. (1972), Etude en microscopie électronique des grains de sécrétion « basophiles » dans les cellules hypophysaires tumorales de la maladie de Cushing. C. R. Soc. Biol. (Paris) *116*, 1591—1595.

Olivieri-Sangiacomo, C., Correr, S. (1973), Ultrastructural features of rat pituicytes in organotypic culture. Z. Zellforsch. *143*, 107—116.

O'Neal, L. W., Heinbecker, P. (1955), The adenohypophysis and hypothalamus in hyperadrenalcorticalism. Ann. Surg. *141*, 1—9.

Orth, D. N., Nicholson, W. E., Mitchell, W. M., Island, D. P., Shapiro, M., Byyny, R. L. (1973), ACTH and MSH production by a single cloned pituitary tumor cell line. Endocrinology *92*, 385—393.

Paiz, C., Hennigar, G. R. (1970), Electron microscopy and histochemical correlation of human anterior pituitary cells. Amer. J. Path. *59*, 43—73.

Pannese, E. (1960), Observations on the ultrastructure of the enamel organ. J. Ultrastruct. Res. *4*, 372—400.

Parakkal, P. F., Alexander, N. J. (1972), Keratinization.—A survey of vertebrate epithelia. In: M. Locke (ed.): Ultrastructure of cells and organisms. New York: Academic Press.

Pasteels, J. L. (1963), Recherches morphologiques et expérimentales sur la sécrétion de prolactine. Arch. Biol. (Liège) *74*, 439—553.

Paterson, J. E. (1948), Cystic pituitary adenomata. J. Neurol. Neurosurg. Psychiat. *11*, 280—287.

Peake, G. T., McKeel, D. W., Jarett, L., Daughaday, W. H. (1969), Ultrastructural, histologic and hormonal characterization of a prolactin-rich human pituitary tumor. J. Clin. Endocr. *29*, 1383—1393.

Pearse, A. G. E. (1950), The histogenesis of granular-cell myoblastoma (Granular-cell perineural fibroblastoma). J. Path. Bact. *62*, 351—362.

Pearse, A. G. E., Noorden, S. van (1963), The functional cytology of the human adenohypophysis. Canad. Med. Assoc. J. *88*, 462—471.

Pease, D. C., Schultz, R. L. (1958), Electron microscopy of rat cranial meninges. Amer. J. Anat. *102*, 301—321.

Peillon, F., Vila-Porcile, E., Olivier, L., Racadot, J. (1970), L'action des oestrogènes sur les adénomes hypophysaires chez l'homme. Documents histopathologiques en microscopie optique et électronique et apport de l'expérimentation. Ann. Endocr. (Paris) *31*, 259—270.

— Gourmelen, M., Brandi, A.-M., Donnadieu, M. (1972), Adénomes somato-tropes humaines en culture organotypique, ultrastructure et sécrétion étudiée à l'aide de leucine tritiée. C. R. Acad. Sci. Paris *275*, 2251—2254.

Pelletier, G. (1971), Classification et physiopathologie des tumeurs hypo-physaires. Un. Méd. Can. *100*, 1779—1783.

— (1973), Secretion and uptake of peroxidase by rat adenohypophyseal cells. J. Ultrastruct. Res. *43*, 445—459.

— Peillon, F., Vila-Porcile, E. (1971a), An ultrastructural study of sites of granule extrusion in the anterior pituitary of the rat. Z. Zellforsch. *115*, 501—507.

— — Pham Hun Trung, M. T., Racadot, J. (1971b), Etude de la morpho-logie et de la sécrétion d'une tumeur corticotrope expérimentale du rat. Rev. Eur. Etud. Clin. Biol. *16*, 79—83.

— Racadot, J. (1971), Identification des cellules hypophysaires sécrétant l'ACTH chez le rat. Z. Zellforsch. *116*, 228—239.

Peña, C. E., Branimir, L., Horvat, B. L., Fischer, E. R. (1970), The ultra-structure of chordoma. Amer. J. Clin. Path. *53*, 544—551.

Pennybaker, J., Russell, D. S. (1948), Necrosis of the brain due to radia-tion therapy. Clinical and pathological observations. J. Neurol. Neuro-surg. Psychiat. *11*, 183—198.

Peters, D., Giese, H. (1970), Detection of DNA in thin sections. In: Proc. VII. Int. Congr. Electron Microscopy, Grenoble Vol. 1.

— — (1971), Elektronenmikroskopischer Nachweis von DNS. Acta Histo-chem. Suppl. *10*, 119—125.

Pflüger, H., Schürmann, P. (1931), Die Hypophysengangsgeschwülste und die Tumoren des zahnbildenden Gewebes, ihre Verwandtschaft im morphologischen Bild und in ihrer Genese. In: P. Schürmann, H. Pflü-ger, W. Norrenbrock (eds.): Histogenese ektomesodermaler Misch-geschwülste der Mundhöhle. Leipzig: Thieme.

Phifer, R. F., Midgley, A. R., Spicer, S. S. (1973), Immunohistologic and histologic evidence that follicle-stimulating hormone and luteinizing hormone are present in the same cell type in the human pars distalis. J. Clin. Endocr. Metab. *36*, 125—141.

— Spicer, S. S., Orth, D. N. (1970), Specific demonstration of the human hypophyseal cells which produce adrenocorticotropic hormone. J. Clin. Endocr. Metab. *31*, 347—361.

Pinkus, H., Mehregan, A. H. (1973), Tumoren der Haut. In: W. Doerr, G. Seifert, E. Uehlinger (eds.): Spezielle pathologische Anatomie. Vol. 7. Haut und Anhangsgebilde. Berlin-Heidelberg-New York: Springer.

Plotz, C. M., Knowlton, A. I., Regan, C. (1952), The natural history of Cushing's syndrome. Amer. J. Med. *13*, 597—614.

Ponté, C., Barry, J., Gaudier, B., Nuyts, J. P., Ryckewaert, Ph. (1968), Modifications de l'hypophyse observées dans deux cas d'hypothyroidie congénitale. Lille Méd. *13*, 675—683.

Poon, T. P., Hirano, A., Zimmerman, H. M. (1971), Electron microscopic atlas of brain tumors. New York: Grune & Stratton.

Popovitch, E. R., Sutton, C. H., Becker, N. H., Zimmerman, H. M. (1970), Fine structure and histochemical studies of choristomas of the neurohypophysis. J. Neuropath. Exp. Neurol. *29*, 155—156.

Poppen, J. L., Packard, A. (1966), Granular cell myoblastoma of the pituitary body simulating a chromophobe adenoma. Lahey Clinic Found. Bull. *15*, 25—27.

Porcile, E., Brye, C. de, Racadot, J. (1964), Données ultrastructurales concernant une tumeur adénohypophysaire humaine. J. Microscopie *3*, 49.

— Racadot, J. (1966), Ultrastructure des cellules de Crooke observées dans l'hypophyse humaine au cours de la maladie de Cushing. C. R. Acad. Sci. Paris *263*, 948—951.

Porte, A., Klein, M. J., Stoeckel, M. E., Stutinsky, F. (1971), Sur l'existence de cellules de type « corticotrope » dans la pars intermedia de l'hypophyse du rat. Z. Zellforsch. *115*, 60—68.

Pour, P., Althoff, J., Cardesa, A. (1973), Granular cells in tumors and in nontumorous tissue. Arch. Path. (Chicago) *95*, 135—138.

Priesel, A. (1922), Über Gewebsmißbildungen in der Neurohypophyse und am Infundibulum des Menschen. Virchow's Arch. *238*, 423—440.

Purnell, D. C., Smith, L. H., Scholz, D. A., Elveback, L. R., Arnaud, C. D. (1971), Primary hyperparathyroidism: A prospective clinical study. Amer. J. Med. *50*, 670—678.

Purves, H. D. (1966), Cytology of the adenohypophysis. In: G. W. Harris and B. T. Donovan (eds.): The pituitary gland. Vol. 1, pp. 147—232. London: Butterworths.

— Bassett, E. G. (1963), The staining reactions of pars intermedia cells and their differentiation form pars anterior cells. In: J. Benoit, C. Da Lage (eds.): Cytologie de l'adénohypophyse, p. 231—243. Paris: Editions du Centre National de La Recherche Scientifique.

Racadot, J. (1964), Reproduction des cellules glandulaires. Biol. Méd. (Paris) *53*, 700—727.

— (1966a), Histopathologie de l'hypophyse. Rev. Prat. *16*, 22—31.

— (1966b), Histologie de l'hypophyse au cours des hypercorticismes. Rev. Prat. *16*, 4127—4134.

— Olivier, L., Porcile, E., Brye, D. de, Klotz, H. P. (1964), Adénome hypophysaire du type « mixte » avec symptomatologie acromegalique II. Etude au microscope optique et au microscope électronique. Ann. Endocr. (Paris) *25*, 503—507.

— — — Droz, B. (1965), Appareil de Golgi et origine des grains de sécrétion dans les cellules adénohypophysaires chez le rat. Etude radioautographique en microscopie électronique après injection de leucine tritiée. C. R. Acad. Sci. Paris *261*, 2972—2974.

— Peillon, F., Decourt, J., Gilbert-Dreyfuss, (1966a), Le problème de la nature des adénomes hypophysaires dans la maladie de Cushing. Sem. Hôp. Paris *42*, 470—477.

— — (1966b), Histologie de l'hypophyse aucours du myxoedème thyroidien primitif. Sem. Hôp. Paris *42*, 482—487.

— — (1968), Modifications histologiques et histopathologiques de l'antéhypophyse au cours de la grossesse. Probl. Act. Endocr. et Nutr. Série *12*, 145—148 (Exp. Scient, éd.).

Racadot, J., Vila-Porcile, E., Peillon, F., Olivier, L. (1970), Structure des cellules dites « basophiles mélanotropes » de l'hypophyse humaine normale et pathologique. Bu. Ass. Anat. (Nancy) *149*, 1095—1096.

— — — — (1971), Adénomes hypophysaires à cellules à prolactine: étude structurale et ultrastructurale, corrélations anatomo-cliniques. Ann. Endocr. (Paris) *32*, 298—305.

Radnót, M., Lapis, K. (1970), Ultrastructure of the caruncular oncocytoma. Ophthalmologica (Basel) *161*, 63—77.

Raimondi, A. J., Mullan, S., Evans, J. P. (1962), Human brain tumors: An electron microscopic study. J. Neurosurg. *19*, 731—753.

Ramsey, H. J. (1965), Fine structure of the surface of the cerebral cortex of human brain. J. Cell Biol. *26*, 323—333.

Rap, Z. M., Zarska, B. (1970), Wysepkowy "myoblastoma granulocellulare" w lejku przysadki mozgowej. (Insular myoblastoma granulocellulare in the pituitary stalk.) Neuropath. Pol. *8*, 121—125.

Rees, J. R., Bayliss, R. I. S. (1959), Cushing's syndrome with pituitary tumor and pigmentation. Proc. Roy. Soc. Med. *52*, 256—257.

Reinhardt, H. F., Henning, L. C., Rohr, H. P. (1969), Morphologisch-ultrastrukturelle Untersuchungen am Hypophysenhinterlappen der Ratte nach Dehydratation. Z. Zellforsch. *102*, 182—192.

Rennels, E. G. (1963), Gonadotrophic cells of rat hypophysis. In: J. Benoit, C. Da Lage (eds.): Cytologie de l'adénohypophyse, p. 201—213. Paris: Editions du Centre National de la Recherche Scientifique.

— (1964), Electron microscopic alterations in the rat hypophysis after scalding. Amer. J. Anat. *114*, 71—91.

— Bogdanove, E. M., Arimura, A., Saito, M., Schally, A. V. (1971), Ultrastructural observations of rat pituitary gonadotrophs following injection of purified porcine LH-RH. Endocrinology *88*, 1318—1326.

Reynolds, E. S. (1963), The use of lead citrate at high pH as an electron-opaque stain in electron microscopy. J. Cell Biol. *17*, 208—212.

Rhodin, J. A. G. (1962), The diaphragm of capillary endothelial fenestrations. J. Ultrastruct. Res. *6*, 171—185.

— (1963), An atlas of ultrastructure. Philadelphia: Saunders.

Richardson, J. F., Katayama, I. (1971), Neoplasm to neoplasm metastasis.—An acidophil adenoma harbouring metastatic carcinoma: a case report. Arch. Path. (Chicago) *91*, 135—139.

Rinehart, J. F., Farquhar, M. G. (1953), Electron microscopic studies of the anterior pituitary gland. J. Histochem. Cytochem. *1*, 93—113.

— — (1955), The fine vascular organization of the anterior pituitary gland.—An electron microscopic study with histochemical correlations. Anat. Rec. *121*, 207—239.

Robert, F. (1973), L'adénome hypophysaire dans l'acromégalie-gigantisme. Etude macroscopique, histologique et ultrastructurale. Neurochirurgie *19*, Suppl. *2*, 117—162.

Robertson, D. M. (1964), Electron microscopic studies of nuclear inclusions in meningiomas. Amer. J. Path. *45*, 835—848.

Roessmann, U., Kaufman, B., Friede, R. L. (1970), Metastatic lesions in the sella turcica and pituitary gland. Cancer *25*, 478—480.

Romeis, B. (1940), Hypophyse. In: M. v. Möllendorff (ed.).: Handbuch der mikroskopischen Anatomie des Menschen. Vol. 6, part 3. Berlin: Springer.

Rose, A.-M., Mennig, H. (1969), Karzinommetastasen in der Hypophyse. Arch. Geschwulstforsch. *34*, 54—61.

Roth, S. I. (1962), Pathology of the parathyroids in hyperparathyroidism. Arch. Path. (Chicago) *73*, 495—510.

— Olen, E., Hansen, L. S. (1962), The eosinophilic cells of the parathyroid (oxyphil cells), salivary (oncocytes), and thyroid (Hürthle cells) glands: Light and electron microscopic observations. Lab. Invest. *11*, 933—941.

Rovit, R. L., Fein, J. M. (1972), Pituitary apoplexy: a review and reappraisal. J. Neurosurg. *37*, 280—288.

Rubinstein, L. J. (1972), Tumors of the central nervous system. In: Atlas of tumor pathology, 2nd series, fascicle 6, Washington D.C.: Armed Forces Institute of Pathology.

Russell, D. S., Rubinstein, L. J. (1971), Pathology of tumours of the nervous system, 3rd ed. London: E. Arnold.

Russell, W. O., Ibanez, M. L., Clark, R. L., White, E. C. (1963), Thyroid carcinoma. Classification, intraglandular dissemination, and clinico-pathologic study based upon organ sections of 80 glands. Cancer *16*, 1425—1460.

Saeger, W. (1973a), Licht- und elektronenmikroskopische Untersuchungen zur sekretorischen Aktivität von Hypophysenadenomen bei Akromegalie. Virchow's Arch., Abt. A, Path. Anat. *385*, 343—354.

— (1973b), Light and electron microscopic studies of pituitary adenomas from patients with acromegaly correlated with the plasma level of growth hormone. In: H. Kulendahl, M. Brock, D. Le Vay, T. J. Weston (eds.): Modern Aspects of Neurosurgery. Vol. 4.—Proceedings of the German Society for Neurosurgery. Amsterdam: Excerpta Medica.

— (1973c), Fine structure of corticotrophic cells and of pituitary adenomas in Cushing's syndrome. Acta Endocr. (Kobenhavn) Suppl. *173*, 28.

Salassa, R. M., Kearns, T. P., Kernohan, J. W., Sprague, R. G., MacCarty, C. S. (1959), Pituitary tumors in patients with Cushing's syndrome. J. Clin. Endocr. *19*, 1523—1539.

Salazar, H. (1963), The pars distalis of the female rabbit hypophysis: An electron microscopic study. Anat. Rec. *147*, 469—497.

— (1968), Ultrastructural evidence for the existence of a non-secretory sustentacular cell in human adenohypophysis. Anat. Rec. *160*, 419—420 (abstr.).

— MacAulay, M. A., Charles, D., Prado, M. (1969), The human hypophysis in anencephaly. I. Ultrastructure of the pars distalis. Arch. Path. (Chicago) *87*, 201—211.

— Peterson, R. R. (1964), Morphologic observations concerning the release and transport of secretory products in the adenohypophysis. Amer. J. Anat. *115*, 199—216.

Santolaya, R. C., Bridges, T. E., Lederis, K. (1972), Elementary granules, small vesicles and exocytosis in the rat neurohypophysis after acute haemorrhage. Z. Zellforsch. *125*, 277—288.

Satyamurti, S., Huntington, H. W. (1972), Granular cell myoblastoma of the pituitary. Case report. J. Neurosurg. *37*, 483—486.

Schechter, J. (1969), The ultrastructure of the stellate cell in the rabbit pars distalis. Amer. J. Anat. *126*, 477—488.

— (1972), Ultrastructural changes in the capillary bed of human pituitary tumors. Amer. J. Path. *67*, 109—126.

Schechter, J. (1973a), Electron microscopic studies of human pituitary tumors. I. Chromophobic adenomas. Amer. J. Anat. *138*, 371—386.

— (1973b), Electron microscopic studies of human pituitary tumors. II. Acidophilic adenomas. Amer. J. Anat. *138*, 387—400.

Schelin, U. (1962), Chromophobe and acidophil adenomas of the human pituitary gland. Acta Path. Microbiol. Scand. Suppl. *158*.

— (1969), Effects of simultaneous thyroidectomy and oestrone treatment on the pituitary cytology in the mouse. Acta Pat. Microbiol. Scand. *75*, 537—544.

Schloffer, H. (1907), Erfolgreiche Operation eines Hypophysentumors auf nasalem Wege. Wien. klin. Wschr. *20*, 621—624.

Schlote, W. (1966), Rosenthalsche „Fasern" und Spongioblasten im Zentralnervensystem. II. Elektronenmikroskopische Untersuchungen. Bedeutung der Rosenthalschen „Fasern". Beitr. path. Anat. *133*, 461—480.

— (1967), Beitrag zum Vorkommen und zu Veränderungen an intracytoplasmatischen Filamenten in Gliomen. Acta Neuropath. (Berl.) *8*, 108—112.

Schmidt, M. B. (1902), Über die Pacchionischen Granulationen und ihr Verhältnis zu den Sarcomen und Psammomen der Dura mater. Virchow's Arch. *170*, 429—464.

Schneider, H. P. G., McCann, S. M. (1970), Release of LH-releasing factor (LRF) into the peripheral circulation of hypophysectomized rats by dopamine and its blockage by estradiol. Endocrinology *87*, 249—253.

Schochet, S. S., Jr., McCormick, W. F., Halmi, N. S. (1972a), Acidophil adenomas with intracytoplasmic filamentous aggregates.—A light and electron microscopic study. Arch. Path. (Chicago) *94*, 16—22.

— Halmi, N. S., McCormick, W. F. (1972b), PAS-positive hyalin in ACTH-MSH cells of man. Structure and presumed functional significance. Arch. Path. (Chicago) *93*, 457—463.

— — — (1974), Pituitary gland in patients with Hurler syndrome. Light and electron microscopic study. Arch. Path. (Chicago) *97*, 96—99.

Scholz, D. A., Gastineau, C. F., Harrison, E. G. (1962), Cushing's syndrome with malignant chromophobe tumor of the pituitary and extracranial metastasis: Report of case. Proc. Staff Meet. Mayo Clin. *37*, 31—42.

Schönemann, A. (1892), Hypophysis und Thyreoidea. Virchow's Arch. *129*, 310—336.

Schultze, W. H. (1914), Tödliche Menorrhagie in einem Fall von Thyreoaplasie mit Hautzelladenom der Hypophyse. Virchow's Arch. *216*, 443—452.

Schurr, P. H. (1966), Pituitary tumours in man. In: G. W. Harris, B. T. Donovan (eds.): The pituitary gland. Vol. 2. London: Butterworths.

Schwidde, J. T., Meyers, R., Sweeney, D. B. (1951), Intracerebral metastatic granular cell myoblastoma. J. Neuropath. Exp. Neurol. *10*, 30—39.

Seemayer, T. A., Blundell, J. S., Wigglesworth, F. W. (1972), Pituitary craniopharyngioma with tooth formation. Cancer *29*, 423—430.

Sekino, H., Nagai, M., Chigasaki, H., Sano, K. (1969), Infundibulo-pituicytoma and granular-cell myoblastoma. Brain, Nerve (Tokyo) *21*, 911—920.

Shanklin, W. M. (1947), On the origin of tumorettes in human neurohypophysis. Anat. Rec. *99*, 297—327.

— (1953), The origin, histology and senescence of tumorettes in the human neurohypophysis. Acta Anat. (Basel) *18*, 1—20.

Shear, M. (1960), The histogenesis of the so-called "granular cell myoblastoma". J. Path. Bact. *80*, 225—228.

Sheldon, W. H., Golden, A., Bondy, P. K. (1954), Cushing's syndrome produced by a pituitary basophil carcinoma with hepatic metastases. Amer. J. Med. *17*, 134—142.

Shiefer, H. G., Hübner, G., Kleinsasser, O. (1968), Riesenmitochondrien aus Onkozyten menschlicher Adenolymphome. Isolierung, morphologische und biochemische Untersuchungen. Virchow's Arch. (Zellpathol.) *1*, 230—239.

Shiino, M., Williams, G., Rennels, E. G. (1972), Ultrastructural observation of pituitary release of prolactin in the rat by suckling stimulus. Endocrinology *90*, 176—187.

— Williams, M. G., Rennels, E. G. (1973), Thyroidectomy cells and their response to thyrotropin releasing hormone (TRH) in the rat. Z. Zellforsch. *138*, 327—332.

Shirahama, T., Cohen, A. S. (1967), High-resolution electron microscopic analysis of the amyloid fibril. J. Cell Biol. *33*, 679—708.

Simonds, J. P., Brandes, W. C. (1925), The pathology of the hypophysis. I. The presence of abnormal cells in the posterior lobe. Amer. J. Path. *1*, 209—216.

Simonds, M. (1914), Über sekundäre Geschwülste des Hirnanhangs und ihre Beziehungen zum Diabetes insipidus. Münch. med. Wschr. *61*, 180—181.

Siperstein, E. R., Allison, V. F. (1965), Fine structure of the cells responsible for secretion of adrenocorticotropin in the adrenalectomized rat. Endocrinology *76*, 70—79.

— Miller, K. J. (1970), Further cytophysiologic evidence for the identity of the cells that produce adrenocorticotropic hormone. Endocrinology *86*, 451—486.

Skorpil, F. (1940), Zur Histologie und Histogenese des papillären Cystadenolymphoms der Parotisdrüse. Frankf. Z. Path. *54*, 181—198.

Sloper, J. C. (1966), The experimental and cytopathological investigation of neurosecretion in the hypothalamus and pituitary. In: G. W. Harris, B. T. Donovan (eds.): The pituitary gland. Vol. 3. London: Butterworths.

Smith, R. D., Northrop, R. L. (1971), Paramyxovirus-like structures in the nephrotic syndrome. Amer. J. Clin. Path. *56*, 97—103.

Smith, R. E., Farquhar, M. G. (1966), Lysosome function in the regulation of the secretory process in cells of the anterior pituitary gland. J. Cell Biol. *31*, 319—347.

— — (1970), Modulation in nucleoside diphosphatase activity of mammotrophic cells of the rat adenohypophysis during secretion. J. Histochem. Cytochem. *18*, 237—250.

Smoler, F. (1909), Zur Operation der Hypophysentumoren auf nasalem Wege. Wien. klin. Wschr. *22*, 1488—1489.

Sobel, H. J., Marquet, E., Avrin, E., Schwarz, R. (1971), Granular cell myoblastoma: An electron microscopic and cytochemical study illustrating the genesis of granules and aging of myoblastoma cells. Amer. J. Path. *65*, 59—71.

— Schwarz, R., Marquet, E. (1973a), Light and electron-microscope study of the origin of granular cell myoblastoma. J. Path. Bact. *109*, 101—111.

Sobel, H. J., Marquet, E., Schwarz, R. (1973b), Is schwannoma related to granular cell myoblastoma? Arch. Path. (Chicago) 95, 396—401.

Soffer, D., Brucher, J. M., Wechsler, W. (1970), Zur Feinstruktur menschlicher Chordome. Path. Europ. 5, 420—441.

Solitare, G. E., Jatlow, P. (1967), Adenohypophysial carcinoma. Case report. J. Neurosurg. 26, 624—632.

Sorokin, S. (1962), Centrioles and the formation of rudimentary cilia by fibroblasts and smooth muscle cells. J. Cell Biol. 15, 363—377.

Spjut, H. J., Luse, S. A. (1964), Chordoma: an electron microscopic study. Cancer 17, 643—656.

— Dorfman, H. D., Fechner, R. E., Ackerman, L. V. (1971), Tumors of bone and cartilage. In: Atlas of tumor pathology, 2nd series, fascicle 5. Washington D.C.: Armed Forces Institute of Pathology.

Sternberg, C. (1921), Ein Choristom der Neurohypophyse bei ausgebreiteten Oedemen. Zbl. allg. Path. 31, 585—591.

Sternberger, L. A. (1967), Electron microscopic immunochemistry: a review. J. Histochem. Cytochem. 15, 139—159.

Stoeckel, M. E., Dellmann, H.-D., Porte, A., Gertner, C. (1971), The rostral zone of the intermediate lobe of the mouse hypophysis, a zone of particular concentration of corticotropic cells.—A light and electron microscopic study. Z. Zellforsch. 122, 310—322.

Stokes, H., Boda, J. M. (1968), Immunofluorescent localization of growth hormone and prolactin in the adenohypophysis of fetal sheep. Endocrinology 83, 1362—1366.

Strada, F. (1911), Beiträge zur Kenntnis der Geschwülste der Hypophyse und der Hypophysengegend. Virchow's Arch. 203, 1—65.

Stratmann, I. E., Ezrin, C., Sellers, E. A., Simon, G. T. (1972), The origin of thyroidectomy cells as revealed by high resolution radioautography. Endocrinology 90, 728—734.

Strong, E. W., McDivitt, R. W., Brasfield, R. D. (1970), Granular cell myoblastoma. Cancer 25, 415—422.

Stutinsky, F., Porte, A., Stoeckel, M.-E. (1964), Sur les modifications ultrastructurales de la pars tuberalis du rat après hypophysectomie. R. C. Acad. Sci. Paris 259, 1765—1767.

Svien, H. J., Colby, M. Y. (1967), Treatment for chromophobe adenoma. Springfield: Ch. C Thomas.

Svolos, D. G. (1969), Craniopharyngiomas.—A study based on 108 verified cases. Acta Chir. Scand. Suppl. 403.

Symon, L., Ganz, J. C., Burston, J. (1971), Granular cell myoblastoma of the neurohypophysis. Report of two cases. J. Neurosurg. 35, 82—89.

Talerman, A., Dawson-Butterworth, K. (1966), Granular cell myoblastoma of the pituitary. Postgrad. Med. J. 42, 216—218.

Tandler, B. (1966a), Fine structure of oncocytes in human salivary glands. Virchow's Arch. 341, 317—326.

— (1966b), Warthin's tumor. Electron microscopic studies. Arch. Otolaryng. (Chicago) 84, 68—76.

— Hoppel, C. L. (1972), Mitochondria. In: M. Locke (ed.): Ultrastructure of cells and organisms. New York: Academic Press.

— Hutter, R. V. P., Erlandson, R. A. (1970), Ultrastructure of oncocytoma of the parotid gland. Lab. Invest. 23, 567—580.

— Shipkey, F. H. (1964), Ultrastructure of Warthin's tumor. I. Mitochondria. J. Ultrastruct. Res. 11, 292—305.

Tani, E., Kawamura, Y., Ametani, T., Handa, H., Imura, H., Kato, Y. (1969), Immunocytochemistry of acidophil granules of human pituitary. Arch. Neurol. (Chicago) *20*, 634—643.

Tashjian, A. H., Jr., Bancroft, F. C., Levine, L. (1970), Production of both prolactin and growth hormone by clonal strains of rat pituitary tumor cells. Differential effects of hydrocortisone and tissue extracts. J. Cell Biol. *47*, 61—70.

Thibaut, F. (1947), Klinik und Histologie der Kraniopharyngeome. Wien. klin. Wschr. *59*, 409—413.

Tillinger, K.-G. (1947), Papillary cystadenolymphoma. Acta Radiol. (Stockh.). *28*, 241—253.

Toga, M., Dubois, D., Berard, M., Tripier, M. F., Cesarini, J. P., Choux, R. (1969), Etude ultrastructurale de quatre cas de leuco-encéphalite sclérosante subaigue. Acta Neuropath. (Berl.) *14*, 1—13.

Tomiyasu, U., Hirano, A., Zimmerman, H. M. (1973), Fine structure of human pituitary adenoma. Arch. Path. (Chicago) *95*, 287—292.

Tönnis, W., Oberdisse, K., Weber, E. (1953), Bericht über 264 operierte Hypophysenadenome. Acta Neurochir. (Wien) *3*, 113—130.

Tremblay, G., Pearse, A. G. E. (1959), A cytochemical study of oxidative enzymes in the parathyroid oxyphil cell and their functional significance. Br. J. Exp. Path. *40*, 66—70.

— — (1960), Histochemistry of oxidative enzyme systems in the human thyroid with special reference to Askanazy cells. J. Path. Bact. *80*, 353—358.

Trier, J. S. (1958), The fine structure of the parathyroid gland. J. Biophys. Biochem. Cytol. *4*, 13—22.

Ulrich, J., Landolt, A., Benini, A. (1974), Granularzelltumor im 3. Ventrikel des Großhirns. Klinische Befunde, Licht- und Elektronenmikroskopie. Acta Neuropath. (Berl.) *27*, 215—223.

Unterharnscheidt, F. J. (1972), Routine tissue culture of CNS tumors and animal implantation. Progr. Exp. Tumor Res. *17*, 111—150.

VanGilder, J. C., Inukai, J. (1973), Growth characteristics of experimental intracerebrally transplanted oral epithelium. J. Neurosurg. *38*, 608—615.

Vanha-Perttula, T., Arstila, A. U. (1970), On the epithelium of the rat pituitary residual lumen. Z. Zellforsch. *108*, 487—500.

VanOordt, P. G. W. J. (1963), Remarks on the pituitary nomenclature. In: J. Benoit, C. Da Lage (eds.): Cytologie de l'adénohypophyse. Paris: Editions du Centre National de la Recherche Scientifique.

Vila-Porcile, E., Olivier, L. (1971), Les cellules follicularies et stellaires du lobe antérieur de l'adénohypophyse du rat adulte. Bull. Ass. Anat. (Nancy) *152*, 812.

— — Racadot, J. (1971), Cellules folliculaires du lobe antérieur de l'hypophyse humaine. Bull. Ass. Anat. (Nancy) *152*, 813.

Vincent, D. S., Kumar, T. C. A. (1969), Electron microscopic studies on the pars intermedia of the ferret. Z. Zellforsch. *99*, 185—197.

Waelbroeck-vanGaver, C., Potvliege, P. (1969), Tumeurs hypophysaires induites par les oestrogènes chez le rat. I. Activité fonctionelle, histologie et ultrastructure. Europ. J. Cancer *5*, 99—117.

Wågermark, J., Wersäll, J. (1968), Ultrastructural features of Crooke's changes in pituitary basophil cells. Acta Path. Microbiol. Scand. *72*, 367—375.

Waggener, J. D., Beggs, J. (1967), The membranous coverings of neural tissues: An electron microscopy study. J. Neuropath. Exp. Neurol. *26*, 412—426.

Walther, H. E. (1948), Krebsmetastasen. Basel: Schwabe.

Warthin, S. A. (1929), Papillary cystadenoma lymphomatosum. A rare teratoid of the parotid region. J. Cancer Res. *13*, 116—125.

Watson, M. L. (1958), Staining of tissue sections for electron microscopy with heavy metals. J. Biophys. Biochem. Cytol. *4*, 475—478.

Wechsler, W., Hossmann, K.-A. (1965), Elektronenmikroskopische Untersuchungen chromophober Hypophysen-Adenome des Menschen. Zbl. Neurochir. *26*, 105—122.

Wegelin, C. (1925), Zur Kenntnis der Kachexia thyreopriva. Virchow's Arch. *254*, 689—709.

Wegmann, H., Landolt, A. M. (1975), (in preparation).

Weibel, E. R., Palade, G. E. (1964), New cytoplasmic components in arterial endothelia. J. Cell Biol. *23*, 101—112.

Welbourn, R. B., Montgomery, D. A. D., Kennedy, T. L. (1971), The natural history of treated Cushing's syndrome. Brit. J. Surg. *58*, 1—16.

Werner, S. C., Stewart, W. B. (1958), Hyperthyroidism in patient with a pituitary chromophobe adenoma and a fragment of normal pituitary. J. Clin. Endocr. Metab. *18*, 266—270.

Whitaker, S., LaBella, F. S., Sanwal, M. (1970), Electron microscopic histochemistry of lysosomes in neurosecretory nerve endings and pituicytes of rat posterior pituitary. Z. Zellforsch. *111*, 493—504.

Whitten, J. B. (1968), The fine structure of an intraoral granular-cell myoblastoma. Oral Surg. *26*, 202—213.

Willis, R. A. (1967), Pathology of tumors. 4th ed., p. 761—763. London: Butterworths.

Wischnitzer, S. (1970), The annulate lamellae. Int. Rev. Cytol. *27*, 65—100.

Wise, B. L., Brown, H. A., Nafziger, H. C., Boldrey, E. B. (1955), Pituitary adenomas, carcinomas, and craniopharyngiomas. Surg. Gynec. Obstet. *101*, 185—193.

Wittkowski, W. (1967), Synaptische Strukturen und Elementargranula in der Neurohypophyse des Meerschweinchens. Z. Zellforsch. *82*, 434—458.

— (1971), Drüsenzelltypen und Hormonlokalisation im Hypophysenvorderlappen. Dtsch. med. Wschr. *96*, 1225—1228.

Worster-Drought, C., Dickson, W. E. C., Archer, B. W. C. (1927), Dyspituitarism of the Lorain type, associated with a pituitary cyst arrising from Rathke's cleft and secondary lesions in the hypothalamic region and ventricles. Brain *50*, 704—718.

Wyatt, R. B., Schochet, S. S., McCormick, W. F. (1971), Ecchordosis physaliphora.—An Electron microscopic study. J. Neurosurg. *34*, 672—677.

Wyeth, G. A. (1934), The histological findings of the hypophysis in cancer. Endocrinology *18*, 59—70.

Yamashita, K. (1972), Fine structure of the mouse anterior pituitary maintained in a short-term incubation system. Z. Zellforsch. *124*, 465—478.

Yohn, D. S. (1972), Oncogenic viruses: Expectations and applications in neuropathology. Progr. Exp. Tumor Res. *17*, 74—92.

Yotsuyanagi, M. (1960), Mise en évidence au microscope électronique des chromosomes de la levure par une coloration spécifique. C. R. Acad. Sci. Paris *250*, 1522—1524.

— Guerrier, C. (1965), Mise en évidence par des techniques cytochimiques et la microscopie électronique de l'acide désoxyribonucléique dans les mitochondries et les proplastes d'allium cepa. C. R. Acad. Sci. Paris *260*, 2344—2347.

Young, D. G., Bahn, R. C., Randall, R. V. (1965), Pituitary tumors associated with acromegaly. J. Clin. Endocr. *25*, 249—259.

Zambarano, D., Amezua, L., Dickmann, G., Franke, E. (1968), Ultrastructure of human pituitary adenomata. Acta Neurochir. (Wien) *18*, 78—94.

Zellner, R. (1959), Die Auswirkungen der Röntgentherapie auf die Odontogenese. Zahnärztl. Welt *60*, 612.

Ziegler, B. (1963), Licht- und elektronenmikroskopische Untersuchungen an Pars intermedia und Neurohypophyse der Ratte. Z. Zellforsch. *59*, 486—506.

Zondeck, B. (1938), Hypophyseal tumors induced by estrogenic hormone. Amer. J. Cancer *33*, 555—559.

Zülch, K. J. (1956), Biologie und Pathologie der Hirngeschwülste. In: H. Olivecrona, W. Tönnis (eds.): Handbuch der Neurochirurgie, Vol. 3. Berlin-Göttingen-Heidelberg: Springer.

— (1960), Über die Strahlensensibilität der Hirngeschwülste und die sogenannte Strahlen-Spätnekrose des Hirns. Dtsch. med. Wschr. *85*, 293—298.

— (1969), Roentgen sensitivity of cerebral tumors and so-called late irradiation necrosis of the brain. Acta Radiol. (Ther.) (Stockholm) *8*, 92—110.

— (1971), Atlas of the histology of brain tumors. Berlin-Heidelberg-New York: Springer.

— Wechsler, W. (1968), Pathology and classification of gliomas. Progr. Neurol. Surg. *2*, 1—84.